MW00584333

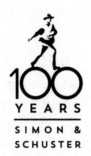

TAKE CARE
OF THEM
LIKE MY OWN

Faith, Fortitude, and a Surgeon's Fight for Health Justice

ALA STANFORD, M.D.

SIMON & SCHUSTER

New York   London   Toronto   Sydney   New Delhi

Please note that names and identifying characteristics of some individuals have
been changed to protect their privacy. All patient names have been changed.

1230 Avenue of the Americas
New York, NY 10020

First Simon & Schuster hardcover edition August 2024

SIMON & SCHUSTER and colophon are
registered trademarks of Simon & Schuster, LLC

Simon & Schuster: Celebrating 100 Years of Publishing in 2024

For information about special discounts for bulk purchases,
please contact Simon & Schuster Special Sales
at 1-866-506-1949 or business@simonandschuster.com.

The Simon & Schuster Speakers Bureau can bring authors to your live event.
For more information or to book an event,
contact the Simon & Schuster Speakers Bureau
at 1-866-248-3049 or visit our website at www.simonspeakers.com.

Interior design by Ruth Lee-Mui

Manufactured in the United States of America

3   5   7   9   10   8   6   4   2

Library of Congress Cataloging-in-Publication Data has been applied for.

ISBN 978-1-6680-0406-7
ISBN 978-1-6680-0408-1 (ebook)

To my readers, young and old,
You are smart enough.
You are beautiful enough.
You deserve to be there.
The abuse was not your fault.
You are not defined by what happened to you.
You are not defined by what you were denied.
Continue to follow your faith,
travel the path not taken,
and take chances on yourself.
You will find that you will not only stand;
you will soar.

Contents

"The story of public health in America wouldn't make any sense if you didn't understand the story of race in America."

—Dr. Ashish K. Jha, Dean of the
Brown University School of Public Health
and former White House Covid-19 Response
Coordinator

Part I

EVERYBODY HURTS

"There is no greater agony than bearing an untold story inside you."

—MAYA ANGELOU

1

PREP

It should have been enough. Saving lives, children's lives, should have been enough. For a long time, it was.

One surgery I performed, on a little girl named Grace, took place right in the neonatal intensive care unit (NICU). We couldn't bring Grace to the operating room, so we brought the operating room to her. Born prematurely at six months, she was just two weeks out in the world. Nothing in her tiny body was ready for surgery. Her entire circulating blood supply would have fit into two shot glasses. Her lungs were fragile as tissue paper, her liver not yet as protected as a full-term newborn's. She had survived this long thanks to miracles of science and the skill of the NICU doctors and nurses caring for her, but her time on this earth was going to end if something wasn't done to repair her gut.

When I explained to Grace's mother what was about to happen, she locked eyes with me. "Take care of my baby," she said. "Make her better." Grace's mom and I were the only Black people present. "I trust you, Dr. Stanford."

"I will take care of her like my own," I said. I meant it. I feel it with every child who comes to me for surgery, every body I cut open. For the next however many hours, Grace would be the most important person in the world to me.

Grace's parents were homeless. That fact likely had something to do with why Grace was born premature. For a mother like Grace's, there would have been little or no prenatal care, no certainty that she would eat anything close to a proper diet. During the months of Grace's gestation, her mother lived under the constant strain of homelessness and uncertainty, her body flooded with stress hormones. There was likely no happy preparation of a baby's nursery, just the shelter where she lived.

Me? I was the doctor, the surgeon with fancy degrees and certificates on my walls reflecting decades of education and career accomplishment. I was well-off, especially by the standards of Grace's mother.

But she and I had two things in common. We were both Black mothers, and we knew what it was like to need and not have. Beyond that, there wasn't much I knew about Grace's mother, her father, their circumstances. There wasn't much I *could* know. I didn't assume they hailed from the same North Philadelphia neighborhood where I was born, though they might have. If it isn't the toughest collection of blocks in the city, it's top five. Barely any green grows there. As a girl, I saw chalk outlines where bodies lay. I knew what it was to be raised by a teenaged, single mother doing her best to manage. A mom who worked multiple low-paying jobs and was gone all the time. I followed the march of roaches on the ceiling above my bed, heard rats scampering across our floor, used food stamps, carried an apartment key around my neck. I knew what it was to be sexually abused by family "friends," with an *s*, and didn't understand why it had happened to me. I knew what it was to be poor and Black in America, and to see adults look me over and drop their eyes and expectations for what I could become. I, too, was once invisible.

It never leaves you, this knowledge. Not ever. No matter how much money I've made, how many degrees and accolades I've collected, how thriving my life: I'll always know what it feels like to need, and to be born into a situation over which you have no control.

When I looked at Grace's mother before I entered the NICU, I saw myself in an alternate universe. Moments later there was no mental space for such ruminating. I rehearsed as I scrubbed. In my mind I saw each operative movement, reviewed each tool of my trade, considered each contingency. I prayed, as I do before every surgery. *God, protect this child. Guide my hands and my mind. Thank you for the privilege of this gift.*

Honestly, it was a miracle Grace had made it this far. We knew *something* was wrong with her, but didn't know exactly what. A child that premature can't be moved to sophisticated imaging machines. But every time the NICU fed her a drop or two of breast milk, her belly distended. Her platelets, the blood cells that help clotting, decreased. Her stool turned bloody and her heart rate slowed. Only the tubes inserted into and coming out of every orifice of her tiny body managed to provide any nutrition and water, and to eliminate her waste. If we let this go on much longer, Grace would bleed into her brain, or her lungs would be damaged. Or both.

Yet there were arguments for waiting. Operating on such a tiny body is risky; you can't afford to lose much blood when you have only two ounces to begin with. Any stray cut, any too-aggressive nudge with my fingers, could tear her liver; any rogue infectious germ could kill her. Maybe, with time, whatever was creating Grace's symptoms would resolve itself. Perhaps she'd gain a little strength and we could operate later.

Every surgeon walks an agonizing line between thinking the solution to every problem is a surgery—it isn't—and being afraid to operate. Surgeons are sometimes accused of having "God complexes." Some do. That can lead to problems. But a good surgeon must be confident and decisive. She can't hesitate. Once she believes in the path, she must move. Skittishness can cost lives just as easily as hubris.

We chose our path. The team and I gathered around this tiny human being, surrounded by equipment on trays and carts, all of us draped in gowns and masks and gloves, me with my headlamp to better illuminate Grace's organs. Aliquots of blood were stored within easy reach. There'd be no time to run to the blood bank if needed.

For a beat or two, the team around Grace was silent but for the hiss of an oscillator pushing air into her tiny lungs, quaking her body with every pump. The violence of forced air can damage such tender lungs, but there was no other option.

"Knife," I said, and the nurse handed me a scalpel with a number 15 blade, a short, curved cutting edge ideal for small incisions. I sliced into Grace's abdomen one finger breadth above her umbilicus—her belly button.

Opening her abdomen, I saw murky brown fluid. Old blood, perhaps mixed with stool. Her intestine was maroon-colored and matted, of questionable viability. Something had happened inside her little belly, and her body had sealed off the dysfunctional parts and let them die.

As gently as possible, I searched Grace's abdominal cavity for pink, living tissue. I found some: a fragment of intestine rested adjacent to the right lobe of her liver, glistening and happy. I had to be careful not to damage her liver, which was already taut and full. Time was running out. The longer the surgery, the more fluid would accumulate in the liver.

Grace's bowel, however, was bonded to other gut organs. I couldn't free it without performing lysis of adhesions, a technique to cut away scar tissue that can bridge space between organs and bind them together. Twenty minutes ticked away as I worked, the hissing oscillator shaking Grace's little body. All the while, more fluid accumulated in her liver.

At last, I managed to free up her bowel, and to palpate the orogastric tube that the NICU had placed in her stomach. I ran my fingers from the tube through her bowel to look for disease. I found it in the jejunum, the middle section of the small intestine. It appeared tan, infected, stuck to the liver. The jejunum was "friable": It easily disintegrated, like wet tissue when touched. That part of Grace's bowel had died. I had no choice but to leave it there and look for other perforations or disease that had led Grace's immune system to wall off and sacrifice this part of her bowel.

As I searched for the root cause of the damage, I found other sections of the bowel, between Grace's stomach and appendix, that were also dead or dying. But some were viable. The operation became one of cutting and assessing the still living sections, removing as much dead tissue as possible, and sewing the remaining living sections back together into one contiguous, though shortened, bowel. I would have to remove her appendix and create an ileostomy, all without losing much of her minimal blood supply.

I let out a sigh at the prospect. This was a lot to ask of the body of a baby who'd been growing for just twenty-six weeks.

I began. Every move, every cut, every stitch, every knot had to be just right. There was no time for second chances or do-overs. The team of nurses, the NICU doc, the respiratory therapists, and I all worked in harmony, our hands and minds singularly focused on saving Grace, step by careful step.

I could not tell you how long this all took. Too long, I thought at the time. Yet Grace's vital signs remained stable. She was a tough girl.

Finally, I created an ileostomy, a passage for stool to leave the body. Too tight and it would block waste; too loose and it would prolapse, or retreat, into the abdomen. The abdominal incision also had to be just right—if I made it too tight, I would wind up creating abdominal compartment syndrome, a condition where the body has difficulty ventilating the lungs fully. I'd suffocate Grace.

There is a moment when the surgeon places the final sutures in an incision at the end of an operation and allows her mind to review what she's just done. *Did I forget anything? Did I do the best I could for my patient? Was my technique the best it could be? Was my inspection thorough? Is my instrument count correct?*

And sometimes, as you finish up, you also wonder if what you've done could ever be enough. As I placed the final stitch to close Grace's small body, I took such a moment. I was amazed at how well she'd tolerated my rooting around inside her. She seemed determined, almost willful. Grace's mother had reminded me a little of myself, and now Grace did, too.

She'd survived the surgery, but she lived without guarantee. More trials stood in her way. The twenty-four- to forty-eight-hour period that followed would be only the first. She would have to withstand constant monitoring by nurses and respiratory therapists. If she scaled that barrier, she would require a long recovery, time to grow and gain strength, then more surgery to reverse the stoma, allowing her to poop through her anus instead of her abdominal wall.

But even if she demolished all *those* obstacles, even if little Grace made it through all that . . . where would she go? Would she and her mother continue to live in a shelter or couch surf? What kind of environment was that for a premature infant with an ileostomy that required close monitoring so she didn't become dehydrated, infected, or malnourished?

I could employ my decades of training and experience, and the others who aided me could use their years of training and expertise, and together we could draw on the accumulated knowledge of a thousand years of medicine, using the latest, most miraculous modern technology to keep Grace alive. But we could not cure the deeper diseases that plagued her and her mother and so many others: injustice, inequality, indifference. And the root cause of these, in so many cases, is one factor.

The color of your skin.

For so long, for so many people, so many of them Black or other persons of color, many of them poor—but not always, not by a long shot—American health care has been a land of broken promises. Or worse.

The Tuskegee syphilis experiment is probably the most notorious example of medical science abusing Black Americans—though relatively few people realize that it ran through 1972—but it hardly stands alone. Louisiana's charity hospitals, the only places Black people there could go for medical care until 1965, were often glorified holding pens for "experimental material"—that is, human beings. Holmesburg Prison, outside my hometown of Philadelphia, was also a source for human experimental subjects, mostly Black, as were prisons all over the country. Henrietta Lacks's cells could be harvested and cultured without a second thought—never mind consent or compensation[*]—because she was a poor Black woman. In 1946, the Hill-Burton Act was passed to help finance the construction of new hospitals and the repair of older ones, but the law decreed segregated facilities, meaning that well into the 1960s the nation's African Americans could not access hospitals that their tax dollars had paid for.

In 1896, Frederick Ludwig Hoffman, a man who influenced a century of thought about health and insurance, wrote *Race Traits and Tendencies of the American Negro*, a landmark of pseudoscientific racism. Negroes, he wrote, were healthy during slavery, but since emancipation had declined due to personal failings like laziness, sexual immorality, and criminality. By Hoffman's account, Black people lacked what many modern-day conservatives would call "personal responsibility." This attitude is still reflected in much of American medicine and public health: If people are sick, it's their fault. Just like—to take one of countless examples—it was the fault of the people of Flint, Michigan, a majority-Black city, when their water supply was contaminated by lead in 2014, a crisis that lasted a half-decade and exposed thousands of children, Black, brown, and white, to high levels of lead. "Flint has the same problems as Detroit," said one Flint public official, who then denounced Black people (using a revolting slur) for not paying their bills, as if that explained the dangerous levels of lead, and the city's horrifying, life-threatening indifference to addressing the problem.[1]

There are reasons why white people born in 1960 can expect to live,

---

[*]A financial settlement with her descendants was reached in the summer of 2023, seventy years after the fact.

on average, seven years longer than Blacks born the same year,[2] just as there are reasons why Covid-19 shortened Black life expectancy by an astonishing four years between 2019 and 2021 (2.4 years for whites)[3], and none of these reasons has anything to do with personal responsibility. They are the same reasons surgical outcomes for healthy Black children are worse than those for healthy white children even when the surgery takes place in the same hospital, for the same condition.[4]

Health care is not apportioned equally in America, and health disparities prove it. Black and brown people have far higher rates of infant mortality. Far higher rates of childhood asthma, and death from it. Higher rates of diabetes, heart disease, and hypertension. Your status in life is predetermined from the moment you are born, perhaps even before that, because where you live, your zip code, which is largely determined by your race, more or less predicts the quality of health care you will receive over the course of your life. Can you imagine your access to lifesaving health care being dependent on your zip code? Your parent's or spouse's or sibling's or child's access? For most of the Black people with whom I grew up, those are not shocking questions.

Almost every African American knows, from experience, the fact of systemic inequity and the broken promise of health care. They've heard family stories of being turned away from hospitals, of doctors not wanting to see them if they're on Medicaid, of being treated with rudeness, of being dismissed and disbelieved—or they've experienced such indignities themselves. For many, hospitals are the place you go to die. African Americans distrust American medicine for good reason: Our health care system has been untrustworthy. And that's true not just for those on the lowest socioeconomic rungs. Even rich, educated African Americans face this mistreatment.

In November 2020, nearly a year into a global pandemic that put a spotlight on the entrenched health care inequities in the United States (and around the world), the American Medical Association finally classified racism as a "public health threat." My reaction: What took you guys so long?

In my home city of Philadelphia and across the nation, the Covid-19 pandemic provided the most unmistakable example yet of hospitals, political leaders, and many civic organizations either failing to consider the needs of the Black community or choosing to neglect those needs. Throughout the pandemic, we saw the racism of low expectations. In Ohio, a state legislator, a doctor, suggested that infection rates were higher among Blacks because they didn't wash their hands thoroughly. In Florida, an official blamed the state's high infection rate on the failure of Black people to be vaccinated—the old "personal responsibility" canard. African Americans, the tired story went, were worsening a public health crisis because they were careless and ignorant. Similar charges were leveled against Hispanic meatpacking workers and low-income white warehouse workers.

Such attitudes reflect the ignorance of leadership. Why were so many more Black people unable to get tested than whites? Supply chain issues and test shortages affected almost all of us. Still, in and around Philadelphia, there was six times more testing in affluent, white-dominant zip codes than in poor, Black-dominant zip codes[5]. A disproportionate number of Black people work nights, or double shifts, or two jobs. Many are less likely to work from home or have the flexibility to take time off, even if only an hour or two, without losing pay. That made it difficult for folks to appear for a test at an appointed time, between nine and five, Monday through Friday. Yet appointments during those times were often required, and often made electronically, so the digital divide favored certain people over others. Even if you found a weekend location, you often needed a referral or script, especially early in the pandemic. Many people did not have a regular doctor (for reasons laid out above), hence no one to write a script for testing. Many people of color were turned away from hospitals—except emergency rooms, where by law they have to take you *in extremis*. It was not just a question of class and wealth: I knew of many friends of friends, Black people of means, with insurance, *good* insurance, who needed a test and guidance, and who were turned away from hospitals. I knew of them because they called me, seeking help, intervention, *something*. Many Covid-19 testing sites in Philadelphia and America were initially at hospitals, not churches or barber shops or community centers.

Some of these barriers to patient health would crumble if the bias were demolished. I am the first Black woman pediatric surgeon trained entirely in the United States. (Dr. Andrea Hayes Dixon is the first Black woman trained in North America; for many years we were the only TWO Black women pediatric surgeons in America.) I am a rare species. Only 5.7 percent of medical doctors in the United States are Black.[6] There are only about 1,600 Black women doctors in the U.S., period, and very, very few of us are surgeons. Of approximately 15,700 surgical faculty teaching in American medical schools, roughly 125 are Black women, less than eight-tenths of one percent.[7]

Do these statistics matter? Absolutely—though I'm chagrined and maybe a little disgusted to admit that until recently even I didn't fully grasp just how *much* they matter. In the spring of 2020, while I was working at a Covid-19 testing site, an older Black woman walked over to our area. We assumed she was there to be tested. "I heard there was a Black doctor here," she said, inspecting me up and down. "I've never laid eyes on one and wanted to see if it was true." I was a unicorn.

There is a long history of second-class treatment of Black people in this country, of regarding Blacks like Ralph Ellison's Invisible Man. We have to be *seen*. The presence of more African American physicians will help to cultivate understanding and upend assumptions.

I am as angry and frustrated as anyone by the inequity in health care and health outcomes. When I've given presentations on the issue— first, as the director for Minority Health and Health Disparities at Temple University's Lewis Katz School of Medicine; then, as founder of the Black Doctors COVID-19 Consortium during the pandemic; later, appointed by President Biden as the regional director (Mid-Atlantic, Region 3) of the Office of Intergovernmental and External Affairs for the U.S. Department of Health and Human Services (please don't be intimidated by the title)—I regularly challenged the clinicians and government officials seated before me to ask themselves: What might we be doing to contribute to these disparities? What could we be doing instead?

There's no shielding our eyes from this. Such unequal treatment ultimately hurts us all—though, of course, some much worse than others. We can't look at the fact of health inequity and simply throw up our hands in helplessness, as if it's beyond fixing.

The poor have always been with us, goes the saying. Those words make it easier to shrug our shoulders as we walk by the beggar in the street. They make it easier to overlook the role of race, too.

But it isn't just poor and working-class African Americans who are subjected to inferior care, who have their needs and complaints dismissed. Growing numbers of Americans have begun to feel that they don't really matter. Far too many don't expect attention and caring, so they don't look for it. They're on their own. They're disposable. Black people have been plagued by this feeling for centuries. For others, it's a newer experience. The United States spends way more on health care, and gets far less in return, than any other wealthy nation. And we rank dead last among our peer countries in overall health care and health outcomes.[8]

What would health equity in America look like? First of all, what *is* it? Health equity (as defined by the U.S. HRSA Office on Health Equity) is the absence of disparities or avoidable differences in health outcomes, such as disease, disability, and mortality, among people from different demographic groups—racial, socioeconomic, geographic, gender. What's the path forward to eliminating disparities in health care and health outcomes in the U.S.?

In the ensuing chapters, I recount my personal and professional story, which I believe illustrates some of the root causes of inequity. You will view the unfurling of my life as a young student who yearned to be a healer, a doctor, a surgeon, then watch things eventually take an ugly turn as Covid-19 overtook the world, America, and my beloved hometown. At the end of the book, I will share my recommendations for actions to address and eventually eliminate many of these health care inequities, because nothing is achieved unless we act, which also means ceasing to do the things we've been doing for so long that have clearly failed. When creating public health programs and policies, our leaders must consider how people live their lives, and where and why they live them the way they do. For example, the catastrophic impact of "redlining" on Black Americans is still felt, almost a century later. In the post-Depression, New Deal era of the 1930s, the United States government created homeownership programs to offer favorable mortgages. Over time, maps were drawn to show the loanworthiness of neighborhoods all over the country; red meant the least desirable, riskiest areas—almost always Black-dominant. By stigmatizing these areas, by considering investment in them to be dangerous, by refusing services to people who called them home: All of that and more erected a ceiling that blocked access, resources, and overall care. This is true for all communities of need, not just Black ones. The crisis in rural health is an example of a similar dynamic. Policies must be created *for the specific community they aim to serve*, not on the basis of the lived experience of the policymakers.

Broken as our system revealed itself to be during Covid, we have a genuine opportunity to make positive, generational change. For all that I experienced during my own personal and professional journey, I feel as if everything I endured prepared me for a role in delivering on a promise, one yet to be kept. My hardships led to perseverance. The stacked odds led to determination. The disappointments led to resourcefulness. I had confidence as a pediatric surgeon, as I helped one child and another and another, yet I felt even more confidence—and hope—as the amazing team I recruited during the pandemic found ways to touch hundreds of lives every day, and the cumulative number grew to the thousands, then tens of thousands, then hundreds of thousands. And counting.

The most important gift we possess is a shared belief that change is possible, that bad can be transformed into good. Grace, the tiny little girl born at twenty-four weeks, just two weeks new to this world, survived that first operation. Five months later I performed a second one on her, to reverse her stoma, and she handled that one beautifully, too. I took care of her like my own. I'm thrilled to report that within the year her parents secured housing for the family.

About a year after that second operation, the world turned upside down. I felt called by the people in my community to take care of them like my own.

My dream? To reach the point where there truly is no difference between "my" and "their."

2

TWO TYPES OF EXPECTATION: LOW AND NO

It is New Year's Eve Day. The fourteen-year-old, nine months pregnant, is shopping downtown at Wanamaker's department store, a Philadelphia institution, looking for an outfit for her baby-to-be. It is mid-morning. The girl came from work and will soon be heading back to work.

She feels a pain, hard enough to force her to hold on to the nearest wall. It's time. At a pay phone she calls one family member, then another, but can't reach anyone: It's the first year her extended family is celebrating Kwanzaa, and New Year's Day is the last night of the holiday. Everyone, including the father-to-be, is out, busy, shopping, or unreachable at work.

Moments later she is outside, hoping a taxi will stop and take her to the hospital. One goes by, then another and another. "A pregnant colored girl in the '70s standing on a corner in Center City on New Year's Eve," she recounted later. "What cab is going to pick me up?"

She doesn't want to get on a bus because it will take too long, so she does what she knows. In labor, she walks gingerly down the stairs to the Broad Street line at City Hall. She will have to take it almost to the end. Race-Vine, Spring Garden, Fairmount. *Please*, she prays, *don't let my child be born on the Broad Street subway.* Erie, Hunting Park, Wyoming. Almost there.

She steps off at Olney and walks to the Einstein Hospital entrance, where they see she's in labor. She screams so much that they sedate her. She is left in a room.

When she wakes, she is no longer pregnant. She is lying in a bed, in a puddle of blood, with no memory of the delivery. There is no baby.

She rises, roaming the hospital halls in search of her child. She sees a scale and can't help herself: She steps on it, curious to see how much weight she has lost. She is fourteen years old, after all, a very recent fourteen.

She continues roaming until someone sees her and tells her the baby—a girl—has been taken to the NICU. It's okay, though, it's okay. They just needed to do for the baby whatever they do, while the new mom—Carolyn is her name—was under.

When mom and baby leave the hospital, they also have to leave home. Carolyn's mom, a divorced single mother, has a rule: Get pregnant and you're out. Carolyn has been unhappy in her home situation anyway. She and her baby are loaded into a cab with some African artifacts her mother insists she take and a can of Heinz vegetarian baked beans, and they move into a $97.50-a-month apartment on 18th Street, near Simon Gratz High School. It's the three of them: new mom, new baby girl, and new dad—just sixteen years old himself. To get public assistance as a minor, Carolyn must be legally emancipated. A state representative helps with that. Until he does, the electric company won't turn on the lights.

Though Carolyn's mom kicked her out of the house, she hasn't abandoned her. Carolyn is good at sewing, so she works in the basement of her mother's fabric and custom clothing store, making clothes for family, friends, even the politician who helped to emancipate her.

She's working, raising a baby, and attending Germantown High School as a sophomore. Five years later, she's pregnant again, this time with a boy. She and the dad break up before he is born.

Because Carolyn is working all the time to support her young family, out of the house by six in the morning and not home until eight or nine at night, her children learn early on that the ER is where you go for health care needs.

Wait, young lady—you came to the ER because you need health forms filled out before you can return to school?

You kids need a physical?

Are you kidding?

Many of the doctors at hospitals all over the country complain, often among themselves, that Black people abuse the system by going to the ER for nonemergent well-child visits. Quite a few of these doctors, along with outsiders, believe that these ER visits prove that Black parents don't care as much about their kids as white parents do about theirs. Or that Black parents are out and about, doing whatever, and don't make the time to bring their child to a proper doctor's office. Some say that if people like Carolyn were older, or married, things wouldn't be so bad for her and her kids. They're probably not wrong there.

But even if you gave her health insurance, the right kind, or a husband, or a job with benefits, it's clear that the variable that predicts bias and poorer health outcomes is out of her control. She is Black.

This time *I'm* the newborn in the story. Carolyn is my mother. This is my life.

On February 21, 1965, assassins murdered civil rights leader and Black nationalist Malcolm X while he addressed a packed audience at the Audubon Ballroom in the Washington Heights neighborhood of New York City. My mother and grandmother watched from the crowd.

The trauma did not dissuade my mother from later activism in Black community organizations in her adopted city of Philadelphia.

She joined a collaborative called the Black Humanist Fellowship. The other mothers and fathers who were part of it would become surrogate parents to me. They often baby-sat when my mom was at high school or working. They helped when my father left for college. They helped potty-train me and teach me to read. My mom believed the community could uplift you, as did my father. We embodied "It takes a village to raise a child." My mother's belief in this principle paid a huge dividend in my life. I attended Nidhamu Sasa—which means "discipline now" in Swahili—an independent, African Free school, right in the neighborhood. The school provided resources and empathy, and it laid a foundation that would serve hundreds of Black students at a time. It felt like home, a haven from the often fearsome reality of my actual home and neighborhood. My teachers and the principal became part of my extended family. My mother remembers me looking happy in library class, hunched over a sheet of paper, trying to write my name for the first time, glad I had only three letters to deal with.

All the students were Black. Everyone who taught me was Black. But it wasn't just the color of my teachers' skin. It was their understanding that society was ready to teach us "Black is bad." They were there to teach us what the world would not. We learned about African kings and queens, and how we were their proud descendants, something I would never have learned about in public school. When the walls of your physical environment are lined with pictures of beautiful, regal Black kings and queens (the posters sponsored by Budweiser, I remember), when you see your own skin hue in these magnificent, powerful leaders who built the Pyramids and made huge advances in mathematics and science and agriculture and economics and technology and art, it does something to you. There was a whole world that came before, a world where African people were living and discovering and improving things, doing just fine and minding their own business before their continent was colonized. That was the Africa that I first learned about in school. Unlike many Black boys and girls, I did not grow up feeling inferior—at least not then. At Nidhamu Sasa we knew our worth. We learned positive lessons about our heritage that you never saw in the general media. These kings and queens had changed the world, and someday we would, too. The ideology I absorbed was forged in service, giving back to your community, lifting it up.

Each one, teach one. He ain't heavy, he's my brother. Reach back to pull up.

The sayings may sound trite, but that was my soundtrack then. It's been ingrained in me ever since.

My name, Ala, is West African. It means "princess of earthly things" or "mother of the earth," depending on whether it's Ghanaian or Nigerian. I don't think I realized how lucky I was to have a name to live up to, to connect with in a meaningful way. To give a child a name with a legacy is a blessing.

At school every morning we recited a pledge, like the Pledge of Allegiance, only it began, "We are an African people. We will remember the humanity, glory, and suffering of our ancestors . . ." We sang a song every morning, like "The Star-Spangled Banner," only ours was called "Lift Every Voice" and began, "Lift every voice and sing, 'til earth and heaven ring, ring with the harmonies of liberty . . ." The flags we flew were red, black, and green. Green for the homeland, fertility, growth. Black for, well, its Black people. Red for the blood shed by our ancestors. A good deal of Black history, at least in our curriculum, focused on much more than slavery. Yes, I learned about the Middle Passage, but also what came before and after.

Back then, in the 1970s, if you were part of anything the white establishment considered Black Nationalism or Black Power, it automatically meant that you were against any "traditional" American ideas and thinking, therefore you couldn't be Christian. If you celebrated Kwanzaa (we did), you couldn't celebrate Christmas (we did that, too). Somehow Christmas was viewed as a white holiday that Black people didn't celebrate. *What?* As young children, my kid brother, Kamau, and I learned about the seven principles honored on Kwanzaa: umoja (unity), kujichagulia (self-determination), ujima (collective work and responsibility), ujamaa (cooperative economics), nia (purpose), kuumba (creativity), and imani (faith). We got a gift (zawadi) on the last day of the holiday. But we had the best of both worlds: Daddy's mom always had a Christmas tree, and I would get a gift from her, and from my other grandma, too. Then again, I was always instructed to hold back opening one of my Christmas presents to be my birthday present, one week later on New Year's Eve day. I thought that was unfair. Kamau, with a March birthday, never had to do that.

Nidhamu Sasa and the Black Humanist Fellowship instilled in me a strong sense of myself as a young Black person, and taught me I was beautiful. But things were never framed as Black versus white. The teachers and community taught me to value myself for who I was and to do the same for others who looked like me. To understand and appreciate where we came from.

I stayed at Nidhamu Sasa from age one until second grade. It was private, and my mom didn't have the money for Kamau and me to be there the whole time, at least not both of us. Kamau stayed longer.

When I was five, shortly before my brother arrived in the world, my family was shattered by my parents' separation. The trajectory of my life followed the path one might expect—at first. Things got even harder for my mother. Now she *truly* was working all the time. She didn't ask for child support; it wouldn't have mattered if she had because for a long time my father didn't have it to give. He was a young Black man in Philadelphia trying to survive. Would it be a trade, college, or a gang and the streets? It seemed like a combination of all three. He had his challenges then. If Kamau and I had even a small stain on our clothes when Daddy came to pick us up, he wouldn't take us.

After she finished high school my mother studied marketing and retail management at the Philadelphia College of Textiles and Science while also working at my grandmother's custom clothing store, Taifa Kufuma. Eventually, my mom landed jobs working for other businesses, in sales and management.

I became like a mother to Kamau. I was a latchkey kid—literally, I wore a key around my neck—and when Kamau started going to school,

I would take him on the SEPTA (Southeastern Pennsylvania Transit Authority) bus, just the two of us. I had started public school, which had woeful resources, and the teachers' expectations for me were either incredibly low or nonexistent.

I know what it's like when people believe in you, and I know what it's like when they don't.

Public school was so different from my previous learning environment. Most of the teachers were white. To my shock, Black children called each other the n-word. The word was used constantly. I knew it could be a term of endearment, but where I came from, we never treated it that way, so we never ever used it. It was straight-up disrespectful. We called each other by our names, names we were proud to have been given.

But at Lingelbach, my new school, my name wasn't a source of admiration. It just set me apart. Other students made fun of it, especially when they learned its origin was African. My teacher wanted me to go by Anna. Why?

"Anna is easier to pronounce," she said.

Seriously? How hard is it to say *ay-LA*?

Kids mocked my short, "4C" hair (the tightest of all the curly hair types). They made fun of my darker skin and strong features, which somehow stood for "not beautiful." They teased me, *African booty scratcher, you're as dark as tar, at night no one can see you unless you smile.* I had come from an environment where I was told I was beautiful, over and over. Why didn't my new classroom walls have posters of dark-skinned African queens and kings, regal and powerful?

On the other hand, I loved the science field trips in third and fourth grades. Being outdoors, armed with a magnifying glass. It was so cool once I figured how to focus the sunlight to burn leaves.

"Ala, what are you doing?" the teacher asked.

"Isn't this neat?"

The other kids were watching.

"Ala, will you please stop setting things on fire?"

Frogs in formaldehyde, all that stuff: just so cool.

Thanks to Nidhamu Sasa, as well as encouragement from my mother, I was instilled with a strong drive to be the best and work hard. I soon learned that my way to more—some would say my escape to a better life—would come from my mind. It was my way OUT. I was eight when I decided I wanted to be a doctor. At first I wanted to be a veterinarian. But my neighborhood was overrun by strays. Even though I was very young, it occurred to me that I would go broke as a vet because no one had money to take their animals to get medical care. Bye-bye, vet career.

Once, on a rare occasion when we went to the local health clinic, I noticed one of the doctors, a very well-put-together Black woman. She seemed happy. She didn't look like most Black women I knew, so many of whom appeared tired, angry, stressed. This woman was different. She seemed Zen and looked pretty and had nice clothes.

Well, shit, what is SHE doing? I thought. *I'll be like her.*

I have many fond memories of my youth, but when I think about walking through the streets of my Philadelphia neighborhood, here are some images that stay with me: stray cats and dogs all over the place, no collars, no leashes. Blood on the sidewalk. Needles. People fighting. The metal grates my brother and I would never walk on because we had heard that occasionally they gave way and kids fell into the abyss. Row houses, one after the other, punctuated now and then by dark alleyways, which Kamau and I would edge away from because we'd heard other tales, about kids getting snatched off the street into those forbidden zones.

Home was not much better. When we didn't have heat in the fall and winter, Kamau and I took turns ironing the sheets in our beds, to keep us warm. We were lucky we didn't burn down the building.

When I was nine, I briefly put my cornet (a small trumpet) down in the school playground to jump rope. It disappeared. I was terrified to tell my mother, thinking that she would have to pay to replace it and that I was going to get a spanking. So I ran away from home—okay, I hid at the end of the fire escape of our third-floor apartment. Only Kamau knew my whereabouts. He brought me peanut butter and jelly sandwiches when our mom wasn't looking. The police came and took a report. I stayed out there until very late, then slept in a friend's backyard. The next day I just came home. I noticed, in the driveway, cars of relatives that I saw only at Kwanzaa time. I knew I was in trouble.

We kept things from our mother not because we were bad kids always getting into trouble, but because we knew how difficult life was for her and didn't want to add to it. I was ten, Kamau five, Mommy all of twenty-four.

It seemed like I was always playing with fire. After burning a spoon with collard greens on it, I scrubbed to get the char off. When that didn't work, I threw it away, praying my mom wouldn't notice. That wasn't the only time I indulged my curiosity about flames. After watching an episode of *The Brady Bunch* in which young Peter is rescued from a fire, I was struck by the way everyone paid so much attention to him. Fluffing his pillow, bringing his favorite foods, asking him if he was okay all the time. I wanted someone to ask me if I was okay, so I took a piece of newspaper downstairs to the first-floor apartment, used a lighter to start a flame, then slid the paper under the door and ran upstairs. My plan? Set the building on fire and escape quickly with Kamau. Mommy would be so happy we were saved that she would make time for us.

I got whooped. We got evicted.

At Lingelbach, the girls with long hair and light eyes were the popular ones. That wasn't me. I was dark with a short Afro. I was smart, but being smart did not make you popular, at least not then. I tried to look like the other girls. Someone—I can't remember who, maybe a friend's mom—straightened my hair with a hot comb on the stove. As soon as my mother saw it, to the tub I went, to wet and wash my hair. (Back then, if your hair was straight, you were trying to be white, meaning you were probably self-loathing.) Just like that, the Afro was back! I was just trying to fit in.

My teacher decided I had a learning disability. Never mind that I did the work. She thought I was slow, in need of remedial help. I was too quiet. There had to be something wrong with me because I kept to myself in the schoolyard, not really engaging with other kids.

But I *knew* how to interact! I didn't because the other kids and I seemed to have nothing in common. I couldn't relate to them. Maybe I felt that what they talked about was trivial. I'm not saying I was right. One way or another, the school felt I needed to be held back.

When my father heard this, he called them in anger. "She's *bored*," he pointed out. "You're not challenging her! So she sits there, not interested!"

He insisted they test me. They finally agreed, and I tested out of third grade. They transferred me to a class for the academically gifted (AG) and mentally talented (MT), which meant that one day a week I got to leave the Philadelphia public school system and go to Drexel University, where I participated in a class for advanced grade school students. One day a week where I could leave my dilapidated neighborhood for a pristine college campus. It was just an eight-mile, forty-minute trip from home, but it might as well have been another planet. A SEPTA token for the subway, one transfer to the el, and before I knew it my world was transformed from one of no expectations to one of no limits.

The curriculum was early childhood education. The instructors were college kids, and there were always a bunch of beautiful toddlers around, but what most impacted me was not so much what I learned there but what I saw. A campus teeming with college students learning, because someday they were going to be something great, make money, have nice cars and nice homes on streets that sparkled. No malodorous garbage all over the sidewalk and stray cats and dogs wandering around. No abandoned cars and buildings. People looking happy, like they didn't have a care in the world, wearing nice clothes, using big words, walking and talking as if they *knew* their future.

Throughout my early childhood, though I had learned about

respect and self-worth at Nidhamu Sasa, I didn't follow every rule. Far from it. I stole from the grocery store—not out of rebelliousness but hunger, literal hunger. When I was nine and Kamau four, we went to the Acme, where I pilfered Tastykakes—and got caught. The police handcuffed me with my arms behind my back and shoved me into a paddy wagon, pitch-black with no windows. I had stolen, yes, but there's something wrong with treating a nine-year-old that way. Kamau had to walk home by himself. God, it hurts just to write those words. At the Broad and Champlost precinct, I telephoned my grandfather, praying that my mother would never hear about this, knowing that that was impossible. Of *course* he told her. They picked me up on Broad Street, both of them. My mother was embarrassed, but it didn't end my shoplifting career. Sometimes I stole Bubble Yum—stealthily removing individual pieces from the pack (not the wrapper), then later putting them all in big Ziploc bags to sell at school for a nickel apiece. I wanted money so I could eat better.

I never wanted to be broke. (Does anyone?) Money or a bus token was a luxury. I was always hustling. My first real job was a paper route: age ten, *The Germantown Courier*. Rolling up the newspapers, encircling them with red rubber bands, hopping on my bike, launching the tubes at front doors.

As independent as I was, I needed go-to people. In fifth grade, at Fitler Academics Plus School, I met one of them, in Miss Johnson's class. Heather was smart, too, but she also managed to be popular. She was tiny and very pretty, with thick, long pigtails, the hair everyone wanted, and fairer skin than mine—not as fair as the vanilla Black girls, more like caramel to my chocolate. Everyone wanted to be Heather's friend.

She picked me. We became best friends. We played hopscotch and double-dutch and giggled all the time. I would tell her everything.

I had other people, too. My mom's mom's mom, Great-Grandma Birdie (short for DeBirdia), was my heart. She was a no-nonsense, cuss-you-out-in-a-minute, drink-you-under-the-table, tell-it-like-it-is kind of woman. She fiercely protected Kamau and me from the time we were itty-bitty. I appreciated how happy she was for me, always, how she made me feel smart and beautiful, reassuring me that I was accomplishing great things, with even bigger ones to come. Others in the family expressed more mixed feelings about her: Some thought she was a drunk who had embarrassed them more than once. But she was my rock. My mom and Grandma were living every ounce of their lives—as they should—but it didn't leave much room for parenting. I needed to feel love, real love, unconditional love, love unsullied by ulterior motives. My dad could have done that—and later he did—but when I needed him most, when I needed him to tell me I was worthy, he wasn't there. He was in college, then busy establishing himself in his career, then in a relationship with someone who commanded all his attention.

All the while, Great-Grandma Birdie was my sounding board, my cheerleading section, my audience of one. A lot of the time that was all I needed. And I had my best friend Heather, who knew the authentic me. Not a whole lot of people saw that person.

3

BREAKAWAY

I could be stupid about boys. "Girl, you boy crazy," Heather told me, and she was right. I had a crush on a different boy every other day. But I was also scared of them. My mother had started talking to me about boys and sex and protection and sex and sex and sex. She taught me about condoms, the Today sponge, birth control pills. As a middle schooler I thought it was all so gross. My mother's grandma had had her mother as a teenager; her mother had had her as a teenager; she had had me as a teenager. "You're gonna break that cycle," she told me. "I don't want you to work as hard as I did. I want you to be in college without children." I was terrified by the possibility of getting pregnant, but still very curious about boys.

Somewhere between Nidhamu Sasa and Fitler Academics Plus School, my self-worth got lost. I could not see my value apart from my peers, apart from my parents, I could not see it when I looked in the mirror. The lack of self-worth stemmed from the change in my school environment, the lack of daily affirmation, and new kinds of interactions with boys (and later men). In middle school, other girls had something that boys wanted, so the boys "sniffed around" and the girls flirted—but I didn't. No looks, no fancy clothes, no big breasts, no putting out; my mom had put fear in me about that, so instead I looked on and watched my friends get notes, knowing glances, an occasional arm around the shoulder, holding hands, sitting together in the cafeteria, walks in the schoolyard, kissing in the stairway. We used to play Catch a Girl, Get a Girl with the boys in the park and playground, but no one wanted to catch me.

The confusion around why and how boys treated me rocked my self-confidence as I entered my teen years, but it did not shake the confidence I had in my intelligence. *That* I could control. Heather and I shared that. As much as we were giddy and silly, we were no-nonsense. We were on the Fitler cheerleading squad for the basketball team. We did steps in the schoolyard, played double-dutch and hopscotch, but we were serious about our books. There were six of us who were thick as thieves, but she and I knew there was more to the world than what was in our neighborhood. We knew that our mind was our way to bigger and better things. That a win for us was a win for our families. She and I were each the glue, keeping everyone together, and we were the problem-solvers when issues arose. We both held that place in our families. That's another way we got each other: We knew the burden we each carried, recognizing the role we played.

Around that time, I started writing "doctor" after my name. I pointed this out to Heather, thinking I'd impress her.

"Look," I said, showing her my expected title. We submitted our names and future professions for our eighth-grade yearbooks, a prophecy. "I'm going to be a doctor."

She laughed. "That don't mean nothin'," she said. "We *all* put doctor next to our name."

We cracked up! She was going to be something special, that was for sure, but not a doctor. Doctor was a very particular dream, and I'd been told by enough people that dreams could become reality. At least one of the mottos written on my classroom wall at Fitler Academics Plus School, Mr. Strub's class, had me believing it:

If it has to be, then it's up to me.

Great-Grandma Birdie had many sisters, and one of them, Great-Aunt Margaret, was married to Rev. S. Frank Emmanuel, pastor of St. Luke African Methodist Episcopal (AME) Church in Harlem, on Amsterdam Avenue and 152nd Street. He and Aunt Margaret were a big part of my childhood, and not just because Aunt Margaret told my grandmother not to terminate her pregnancy (a fact my mother would not learn until months before Aunt Margaret died). She told my grandmother she would help raise my mom, and she did.

Aunt Margaret was the opposite of my Great-Grandma Birdie. Margaret was prim and proper, every hair in place, a dutiful first lady. She had a beautiful smile and glowing skin, which she kept smooth and youthful thanks to good old Vaseline. Margaret loved us and cared for us with what energy and time she had left after caring for Uncle Frank. He was the focal point, as he should have been.

Every summer during my childhood and adolescence, my mother put me on the bus to travel up to New York for a couple of weeks. I'd go at different times—sometimes for Easter or other holidays, or just for the weekend for Sunday services.

I loved staying in the parsonage, all the cousins running around the house. We ate so well. Aunt Margaret would make breakfast, something I was unaccustomed to in our home. In Philadelphia, I was the one who got breakfast ready for my brother and me every morning; my mom was up and long gone to work by that time. In the parsonage, Aunt Margaret would cook eggs and bacon and sausage and rolls and pancakes and grits with butter. It was like living in a restaurant. I'd come downstairs to the basement and my Aunt Margaret, her hair pinned and tied up, would have all the food prepared. Uncle Frank would eat first, then retreat to his study, and then we would all get to eat. No one went hungry. I can't remember a single Greyhound trip home where I didn't have a brown paper bag filled with a piece of cake or sweet potato pie.

After Sunday breakfast, we'd get dressed and walk across the parking lot, past my uncle's purple Fleetwood Cadillac, and enter the church. No one could look at us funny for taking up the first few rows because that was our Uncle Frank up there preaching. After the service, the whole extended family, invited guests, preachers and their spouses and children would head downstairs to eat a second time. The women of the church cooked incredible food, everything in big bowls and on enormous platters. We'd sit at a gigantic table with "the First Lady," my Great-Aunt Margaret, at one end of the table and Uncle Frank at the other, leading us in prayer before we all ate, family-style.

It was there that the religious seed was planted. I hadn't been taught about being Christian by my mother (who is now devout) or my father. My relationship to Christianity started with those visits to Harlem, listening to my uncle preach. The church, I came to see, holds a central place in Black life unlike any other. It is the anchor. And Uncle Frank was powerful. All these people followed him. I was surrounded by lots and lots of Black folks, but this was not the Black Power that had enveloped me in my first school. This was something different. This was Christianity. I felt its fellowship, passion, strength, and love. I figured, *Well, shucks, Uncle Frank must be saying something important if everyone is acting this way . . .* I started to believe. When I opened my mind to God's presence, my eyes began to see all the ways in which He moved in our lives.

So many things about those New York visits affected me. I remember sitting in the room across from Uncle Frank's study, which overflowed with books. Great wooden partition doors closed him off from the rest of the world. I spent hours on a big green couch in the neighboring room, which had a TV and a white radiator, knowing that he was right next door reading and thinking and writing, and that whatever he was doing in there enabled him to get up in front of hundreds of people and make them scream and shout and sing and sway until some of them passed out from such intense joy. He refueled them for whatever they might encounter throughout the week. But all the magic started in *that* room. I remember his enormous Bible, bigger than any I had ever seen. Once, when I was flipping the pages, my aunt told me not to mess with it.

I also learned more surely that life had a beginning and an end. My cousins and I were once running through the sanctuary on a week-day. As we bolted down the center aisle, a body lay in an open coffin beneath the pulpit. It stopped us in our tracks. We had not yet been formally introduced to death and dying, and it made me think about what happens when life leaves our body, and other questions that only faith can answer.

I tried to incorporate into my life the teachings I was learning. A few years later, after returning home from a weekend in New York, I told my high school boyfriend, "You know, I can't be intimate because I'm following God's word."

"What are you talking about?" he replied.

"I can't have sex."

There was a long pause. "What are you talking about?" he repeated, crushed.

I loved what I got from those trips to New York, a sense of com-munity, service, family—of *love*. And I endeavored to make sense of the key religious ideas: forgiveness, grace, gratitude, humility. Like, why is there a God *and* Jesus? *And* the Holy Spirit? Which one am I praying to? How come some people say, "Jesus forgave me for my sins"? How do they know? Why is this person next to me shaking violently? What does it mean when someone has the Holy Spirit? I'm sure lots of adults struggle with these and similar questions, and I'm sure lots probably don't even think about them that deeply. And when you're a kid, maybe it's even harder to understand. But if I was going to believe, I had to understand what it meant to surrender, and to say that I wanted to be forgiven, and to believe that Jesus died for my sins.

Later, when I was a surgical resident, and I knew each day was going to be long, hard, and exhausting, I recited Psalm 91 to myself in the morning as I walked into the hospital. Why that one? Because its message is that God will protect you from whatever comes your way. When your enemies come toward you, He will shield you. It reminds us to have faith and walk in God's word.

In middle school I began participating in oratory contests. (I still have my third-place plaque somewhere.) The Reverend Dr. Martin Luther King Jr. was our inspiration. On MLK Jr. Day, my class held contests to see how many "goal words" each student could work into their speech. That's the way that many of us overcame a fear of public speaking. We gained confidence in expressing ourselves, and learned that if what we had to say was truly powerful, it shouldn't be written just to be read, but to be read aloud, to an audience of listeners. I was inspired to write an op-ed for our local paper, the same one I delivered around the neighborhood, on why it was important to keep our streets swept clean, to instill a sense of pride in place. Despite the occasional frustrations I had at school and at home, I was finding my voice.

Then someone took it from me.

He worked for the city. He started to hang out near where my friends and I did, and we got to know him well enough that I introduced him to my mom. I thought she would like him.

Unfortunately, she did. He started spending lots of time at our place. After a while he began abusing me sexually, touching my body in places no man should touch a child.

Then I got a reprieve. When I was in eighth grade, my mom got promoted at Kmart to manager and had to relocate for her new position; she left ahead of us to get things settled. My brother and I moved in with my dad and his girlfriend. Things were strict, and she didn't want us there, but for me it was a welcome change.

We followed my mother's positions and promotions wherever they took her, to towns where we knew no one. During that eighth-grade year I was accepted to Central High School, one of the best high schools in Philadelphia. It was the first year it would be co-ed. But right after middle school graduation my mom came back to get us and bring us back with her, to Lockport, New York, outside of Buffalo. At least I remained safe, away from the child molester.

Well, I *thought* I was free of him.

Lockport was an itty-bitty, racist town, complete culture shock. Growing up in Philly I rarely saw white people besides public school teachers, and suddenly we were in a place that was about three-quarters white. It wasn't as if there were *no* Black people around, but for the first time we stood out, and not in a way you'd want. No person of color was in a position of authority. I often felt I was looked at *only* as a Black person, so I (as well as every other Black person around) represented a stereotype—whatever that might be, academically or culturally or socioeconomically—of every Black person in America. Many of the white folks in Lockport were thrown when the reality of a Black person, namely me or my brother or my mother, contrasted with their expectation. It just did not compute. The town seemed to believe Black youth could only ever belong to one of two categories: athletes or criminals. No way could we be the smart kids. At times the racism was overt. I heard the n-word a lot there, too, only this time it was frequently white people aiming it at Black people; it came from young kids, older folks, across the board, as if it was a thoroughly acceptable part of the vocabulary. If I made friends with a white kid, they were called an n-lover. For a while I didn't have many friends there.

It didn't help when my classmates, white and Black alike, heard that I was from Philadelphia. The city's image had recently been tarnished by a truly disturbing national news story: In May of 1985, the Philadelphia Police Department, under the leadership of Mayor Wilson Goode, bombed a house occupied by MOVE (an organization focused on Black liberation and a back-to-nature lifestyle). The Philadelphia Fire Department allowed the ensuing fire to burn, destroying dozens of neighboring homes. Eleven people in the MOVE compound died, including five children.

The reaction from some Lockport kids? "You're from that city where the mayor dropped a bomb on Black people."

And it *really* didn't help that I still got into occasional trouble. I wanted the stuff that other kids had. I tried to shoplift a popular boombox (yes, the whole thing) from a store that, to make matters worse, was a competitor of Kmart, my mother's employer. Naturally, I got caught. They called my mom at work. She showed up, crying and broken. "I'm trying so hard," she said. "I don't know what else to do." This time, seeing that disappointment, hurt, and embarrassment in her eyes put an end to my criminal career.

I would have to learn how to earn what other people had, even if I had to work harder than they did to get it.

And then my mother invited him to come visit us in Lockport.

Our time in upstate New York wasn't all bad. I made some good friends, including Claudette, who I could be real with. I made more friends when I joined the school track team. Running fast came naturally to me, something I had learned back in Philly, and it was the one sport that everyone could participate in. You didn't need a ball, a special court, or a field. You might need sneakers, but for some of us even that wasn't a necessity. Or we shared sneakers. Really, you just needed a street and for someone to say, "On your mark, get set, go!" Many of us did track because the money our parents were asked to invest in it was slim to none. In high school, I did the 100-meter hurdles, the 400-meter hurdles, and the 4x400-meter relay. My mom would come to meets and everyone knew which runner she was pulling for. From the sidelines she would scream her head off and often race down the track alongside us, as if she expected to keep up. Once, early in my running career, I was leading the pack when I heard my mother cheering for me. Stupidly, I looked back, a reflex, to my mother shouting my name. I got passed and ultimately, humiliatingly, lost the race. I never looked back again.

• • •

Then Kmart asked my mother to move again, so we did, this time to South Plainfield, New Jersey, where I would spend the last two years of high school. Though we were being upended one more time, I was glad to get away from him.

But she invited him to visit us in our New Jersey home, too.

In South Plainfield I studied hard, still ran track (now ranked in the state), and listened to lots of Whitney Houston. I'd become more interested in dating. There weren't that many Black boys around; those that were seemed more into white girls. My first real boyfriend was white, and he didn't look at me as if I were Black. But it bothered me that he was white. I worried that Black people would look at me sideways and think I had betrayed my race. Dominic was Italian, and I liked him a lot. He had a mom and a dad and they all lived in a house. He was fine with public displays of affection, but they made me uncomfortable, which bothered him. At some point later in the school year I kissed another boy. No one saw it. The only evidence was what I wrote in my diary, that I wished I had met that boy first.

Dominic read my diary. There were things in there meant for me and God only. I already carried around a deep sense of having been violated, and here was another betrayal, a different kind, but one that cut me deeply. In the parking lot behind our apartment, Dominic confronted me as I reached the bottom of the steps. He was livid about what he had discovered, but he expressed no remorse about how he had discovered it. He punched me in the stomach, hard enough to knock me to my knees. As I labored on the ground, I remember looking up and noticing that the shingles on my building were pale green, and I could see my mom's old black car parked in its space with its matte finish—not because it was cool like today's matte cars but because it cost too much to repaint it. It was light outside. Dominic yelled at me some more while I remained doubled over, then he got in his car and drove away.

I thought I deserved it. When I speak to high school girls now about career choices, making good decisions, and intimate partner violence, I share that story. So many of them can relate from personal experience or that of friends. I reinforce that it's never okay for someone to abuse you verbally with words or physically with violence. But when I was a teenager, this was simply a continuation of abuse that I had come to accept, tuck away, and smile through. Did I know this was not supposed to happen in relationships? No. Why would I? I'd never seen a truly functional one.

In November of 1986, the fall of my junior year, I went back home to see my mother's father's mom. I liked taking the bus from New Jersey to Philadelphia to see family. I loved being sprawled on the floor of my Great-Grandma Brame's living room, watching TV on one of those big brown television sets that look like furniture. One day, I sat there watching the Oprah Winfrey show. The episode featured children my age, some younger, some older. They were being interviewed by a man—a prosecutor, but I didn't know then what that was. Each of the children had been sexually abused or molested. One by one, they told the man about another man, or men, who had abused them. Were the kids witnesses in a trial? I don't recall because I focused on one thing. The children were now sitting with Oprah, and she was saying, *It's not your fault.*

It was the first time I had heard anybody talk about that experience, one that I was living through myself.

More than once.

The first was a bus driver. He lived in the West Oak Lane section of Philly. I remember his name. He dated my mom for a couple of years. He abused me when we lived on Blakemore Street, while my mom was asleep. We slept in the same room, she and I, so part of me couldn't believe what was going on. I started wearing tights to bed, hoping they would serve as a deterrent and he wouldn't pull them down. I slept on a mattress on the floor, and I took the grate off the box fan to put a kind of wall around me. He walked into it once, and I know the blades hit his leg, but it didn't stop him.

I didn't tell her. I was doing all the things I could as a kid to say something without saying something.

Now, sitting on the floor of my great-grandmother's living room, transfixed by what was playing on the TV set, I felt comfort to hear a grown-up say what Oprah was saying. I had never felt I could talk about what I'd been through, and here was the most famous woman in the world saying things I wanted to hear. *It isn't normal. It's not okay. You're not dirty. This should never have happened. There is nothing wrong with you. It's not your fault.* Oprah said that I mattered. Her words were not the words of Jesus. She did not perform a miracle. But I felt some reassurance. I had value. I needed that as a child. All children who've been through trauma need it. Comfort and reassurance and positive messages were sometimes in short supply where I grew up.

Then Oprah said that it had happened to her, too.

There would be no instant cure for me. There would be no true change until much later in my life. Nor would the change happen all at once. It would happen in small moments, like this one, sitting on Great-Grandma Brame's floor, watching Oprah. A bit at a time. I got a glimpse of what I was looking for. It *wasn't* normal. It *wasn't* okay.

In New Jersey I had a bedroom door that locked, but I still preferred to be out of the house. I became increasingly focused on my independence. And for that I needed money. Throughout my childhood, I had always gotten the same answer whenever I asked for money, so eventually I stopped asking. I knew how bad it made my mom feel to say no. I figured out how to earn my own. As soon as I could get working papers, I landed a job at Burger King. I did everything there—flame-broiling burgers, working the fryer, putting apple pies in the oven, refilling the fountain. With the money I made I bought running sneakers, track spikes, a prom dress with the crinoline slip to make it puffy. I learned to drive my mom's car but still rode everywhere on the bike my father had bought for me, back and forth from home to Burger King to school to track practice.

Another plus to working at Burger King: I could bring food home for Kamau and Mommy, especially since I often worked the closing shift and they didn't want us to throw away food. (Today, I bet it's much stricter.) My next job was as hostess at TGIF's, which paid a little better. Now and then someone would slip me a ten and whisper, "Hey, can you get us a table sooner?"

I was enterprising. I earned enough to pay for a lot of the things I wanted. But my No. 1 goal was getting into college. (Later, when I took out my student loans for college—me, not my parents—I paid them off myself.) I needed equally to excel and to get away from home.

I asked my high school guidance counselor about the prerequisites I would need in college to get into medical school. He looked like a nice man. But when he heard what I dreamed of doing with my life, he told me I was "overreaching," that "medicine might be a little too much" for me. This again? Expectations for me and people who looked like me apparently came in three flavors: low, lower, lowest. He paused. "I'm not sure you're medical school material. I'm not sure you have the aptitude. Maybe community college?"

Forget how demeaning his recommendation was. The bigger point was . . . he didn't even know me! I had transferred in for eleventh and twelfth grades. And if he didn't know me, then how the hell could he know what I was capable of? He treated me like he probably treated every other Black kid.

I made a vow to myself: From then until college acceptance, I would ignore the guidance counselor and focus instead on what *I* believed.

I possessed a huge desire to learn, something my mother and father and family had always encouraged. Before our first move, I went to the Philadelphia Free Library on Green and Chelten nearly every day after school. Now, as a high school junior, I needed to get a good SAT score. I was never a good standardized test-taker. I studied dictionaries to improve my vocabulary and came across so many words I had never seen and had trouble pronouncing. Egalitarian. Meritocracy.

Subsumed. Menial. Perfunctory. If your parents are in school when you're in school, or you're not surrounded by people using a certain vernacular, no way you're hearing words like "loquacious" or "taxidermy" in your household. I took the SAT once and bombed, then a second time so I could crack 1000, which I did, barely. (As close as Kamau and I were, we obviously had different aptitudes. He topped 1500 without studying. I was happy for him. God gives us all something and none of us gets everything.)

When it came to actually applying to college, it all fell to me. I frequented the local Barnes & Noble because they had books on how to get into college. I devoured the information in them until I'd saved enough to buy them. I also inhaled the books in the high school guidance office. I filled them with Post-its. I made out all my applications. I paid for all my applications. I was still a Pennsylvania resident (my dad lived in Philly) and had my heart set on Penn State, where I could pay in-state tuition. I applied to Rutgers, too, and the week of Thanksgiving senior year I received their acceptance letter, which was thrilling. But then I got into Penn State and that was that.

Another reason I chose Penn State: My cousin Christophe was a graduate, and at the time he was an anesthesia resident at Hahnemann University Hospital, the teaching hospital for Drexel University. He was the only person I actually knew who was even close to becoming a doctor—except for the well-dressed Black woman in the clinic who'd sparked my dream years ago. *Okay, if Christophe went to Penn State, then I'm going to Penn State. I'm going to do everything he did, and maybe that will ensure my becoming a doctor.*

I sent a money order (I didn't have a bank account) to Penn State for the first tuition payment. I had a map of the university's twenty-four campuses and chose Behrend, near Erie, in the very northwest corner of the state, because it was furthest. I was closer to Canada, Cleveland, and Buffalo than to Philly.

My mother couldn't have been prouder—and not just of me but also for what she had accomplished. She had every right. "All those people who live in those big houses up on the hill," she said to me and Kamau, who later graduated from Howard University and matriculated at law school there, "most of them weren't single-parent households. Most of them had all the shit. They have all the money in the world, and some of them, their kids are all screwed up. And here I am with hardly nothing, and look at you guys. Look at you! Sometimes money doesn't bring success. Or happiness. Or anything."

I got a partial scholarship, which was especially nice because it meant that when I walked across the stage at my high school graduation, I got called out for my degree *and* the award. I was glad for my parents—for both the money and the pride.

The summer before I left for college, I worked at Kmart. They carried merchandise I would need for freshman year—rug, microwave oven, sheets, toiletries—and they offered an employee discount. They also let us put items on layaway. I could have my stuff sit there all summer while working to pay for it.

In the fall, my mom dropped me off at Penn State-Behrend. I was seventeen. Through her tears she gave me a Bible. Later I found the $50 bill she had slipped into its pages. "Don't cry, Mommy," I said. "I want to be here. You can go home. I'll be just fine." Her nest was empty because Kamau was living with our dad by then. I was sorry to leave my brother behind. He was still just a kid. But I needed to get the hell out of there.

4

COLLEGE AND CADAVERS

My first year of college meant I was one step closer to achieving my dream. I could explore, I didn't have to ask permission. For obvious reasons I was happy to get out of the house. I was learning how to prepare for college science classes. To study and work my way into med school. But I was also a kid who wanted to have fun and express herself.

Freshman year we were allowed to paint a mural on the dorm hall wall. They even gave us art supplies. My roommate didn't want to paint so I had the entire fifteen-foot by fifteen-foot wall to myself. I painted a red, black, and green flag with the sun on top of the flag, under a Langston Hughes quotation: "Beautiful also is the sun; beautiful also are the souls of my people." For the rest of freshman year, that was the first thing I saw when I opened my door. It was a happy callback to my classrooms at Nidhamu Sasa and the wall posters of kings and queens.

I took great pleasure in being a Penn State "Lion Ambassador." You didn't just become one; you had to meet eligibility criteria, apply, hope for an interview, and be selected. It was an honor on campus. Some folks called us Lion Ambassadors nerds; maybe we were, but I loved it. Among other things, our responsibilities included providing tours for prospective students and accompanying dignitaries visiting campus. I was fortunate enough to meet Julian Bond, the civil rights leader and later chair of the NAACP, and Shirley Chisholm, the first Black woman elected to the U.S. Congress. I got to attend a dinner honoring writer Alex Haley, author of *Roots* and coauthor of *The Autobiography of Malcolm X*. I also liked the Lion Ambassador uniform: khakis, white shirts, and Nittany Lion bow ties. I enjoyed being a part of something.

The Penn State-Behrend campus didn't have a women's or men's varsity track and field team, so I created one. I put up flyers to recruit athletes. There were lots of replies. I had to find an advisor. I had to find out which meets we were qualified for, then I had to order uniforms. I didn't realize it at the time, but I was learning how to build an organization from the ground up.

Technically, we were a "track club," but we competed at roughly a Division III level, against nearby schools like Clarion, Case Western Reserve, and University of Pittsburgh-Bradford. I won the occasional race, but for me it was about more than winning: Running was part of my identity, my escape in high school, a time I felt peace.

(Years later, when I gave the commencement address at Penn State-Behrend, I was acknowledged for starting their running program, which had become an NCAA Division III varsity track and field program for men and women, with a beautiful all-weather track that hosts track and field meets. And it all started with eighteen-year-old me!)

My academic performance was divided. I wasn't a straight-A student. But I was determined. If I missed a question on a test, I wanted to understand why. I began to realize that just comprehending the information was not enough. I had to be able to answer questions correctly. I had to learn how to take a test. Who knew that was a thing? As my classes became harder, there wasn't enough time to run *and* study, and since I couldn't envision a career as an Olympic athlete, it wasn't a difficult choice.

My friend group was like the United Nations, but at times I felt as if I was part of two worlds. I had great friends who were Black and great friends who were white. (And great friends who were neither, and great friends who were both.) At a club hockey game sophomore year there was a lone Black player, and some idiot fans singled him out: Whenever he had the puck—the black puck—on his stick, they started chanting, "Puck, go home! Puck, go home!" Horrible as it was, no fans booed, no arena staff objected to the racist taunts. No coaches or refs did a damn thing. I imagined what the player felt like, with an audible batch of fans chanting that garbage. Trying to make him feel like shit because of his skin color in an arena of people screaming in unison. I wrote an article in the Penn State newspaper arguing that saying nothing about obvious racism is akin to condoning it. Today we would call it complicity.

Nor was I quiet about more thinly veiled racism. I was quoted in the *Daily Collegian* for a story about course diversification. The university, to its credit, announced a call for curricular diversity. Others countered, advocating instead for "voluntary change rather than imposed alteration of university curriculum." One student Senate member said that "if the need for diversity were real, students would voluntarily take courses in minority studies and faculty members would integrate the curriculum on their own." To me that sounded pretty clueless. I replied that "if curriculum diversity were working, we wouldn't be here discussing it today." It made sense to me then that understanding the plight and culture of others was necessary for empathy. Later, as a surgeon and then especially during the pandemic, I would come to understand that so much more profoundly.

College was a full life, but from the start I never took my eyes off the prize of becoming a doctor. To me, that's what college was for: to major in pre-med so I could ace my MCAT (Medical College Admission Test), apply to medical school, and get that golden ticket acceptance letter.

Studying for my pre-med courses was where I most acutely felt my disadvantage. Frankly, it's where the differences between my culture, experience, and socioeconomic status and that of many of my class-mates were on full display. Unlike them, I had no brother, sister, parent, uncle, or aunt to tell me how to study, to provide study materials they had used. I was pretty much on my own. Many of the undergrads aim-ing for med school came from generations of doctors; they had parents who sometimes even went to the particular medical school their kids wanted—even planned and expected—to attend. They had support coming out their ears. Most of them came from two-parent house-holds. If they had campus jobs, it usually wasn't to pay part of tuition. For me, work-study was real. That's how I paid tuition, not how I bought clothes or incidentals. Every semester I wondered if I would have enough to pay the minimum tuition. Would I get the money submitted before the deadline when a penalty could kick in? Would I get a refund? Would I be too exhausted to study after working a long shift at the job I needed to pay for books and food? How much harder would I have to study or catch up on vocabulary words for the MCATs because I wasn't taught those words in high school nor heard them at home?

Many of my fellow students—more often than not white—didn't have to ask any such questions. They could focus, pure and simple. What a gift. Each step laid out before you.

Okay, now I'm pre-med.

Okay, now I'm a medical student.

Okay, now I'm an intern.

Okay, now I'm a resident.

Okay, now I'm a board-certified doctor.

In the spring of my sophomore year, a guidance counselor alerted me to a summer "health professionals" prep program at Harvard. Its goal was to help underrepresented students prepare to be doctors. Per-fect! I applied and got in. My father drove me to Cambridge, Mas-sachusetts.

It was a transformative summer.

There were Black kids everywhere. And Latino kids. Kids from all over the U.S. Some were from Historically Black Colleges and Universities, some from the Ivy League. Someone had seen a spark in each of us, and here we were, about two dozen in all.

The classes were conducted at Harvard Medical School. One of my classes was gross anatomy, where I first laid eyes on a cadaver (not a corpse in a coffin). I felt strong; I was not going to pass out; I was thrilled to think I was seeing what the med students saw when they examined dead bodies, and that one day I would do this as part of my job. I noticed the nail polish on the fingers of one of the cadavers, and it made me pause, recognizing that this was once a living, breathing person. Few things make you appreciate life like looking at a corpse. It is humbling. We learned about the organ systems by examining those of the deceased; if a person had had lung cancer, you'd see black lungs or a big yellow tumor in the center, or both. If there was metastatic spread in the abdomen, you could see the disease.

We took classes in chemistry. We took lots of practice MCATs. I got a summer job because there were things I wanted—in particular, a Harvard Medical School sweatshirt. At the Harvard Coop, the students' everything store, thumbtacked flyers advertised summer jobs, and I yanked the little paper tabs with phone numbers at the bottom. I got a job pulling weeds in someone's yard, which paid a decent eight bucks an hour. I cleaned houses, which I hated because it made me feel like someone's maid. But I saved enough for the sweatshirt, which cost $50, a lot of money back then. (I still wear that gray Champion sweatshirt, with crimson lettering and the caduceus running down the center—a staff with wings entwined by two serpents, the symbol for medicine.)

As important as what we learned in our classes was the experience of just hanging out—at meals, at night, walking around Harvard Square—and talking about ourselves, what it was like at each of our colleges, our thoughts and hopes and dreams. We put on a talent show. We formed bonds that seemed as if they would last.

Everything I needed to know about getting into medical school I learned that summer. They taught us how to write a personal statement. I needed help on test-taking, so they advised me to take an MCAT prep class when I returned to Penn State my junior year. They gave me a roadmap. They advised me *not* to major in pre-med but biology. Why? For one, the bio curriculum was more well-rounded than pre-med. For another, and more importantly, a bio major gave you a better Plan B in case you didn't get in anywhere. "If you're a pre-med major," they told us solemnly, "how are you going to get a job if you're not in medical school?"

That summer I liked feeling smart. I liked knowing that the grades I got in Harvard science classes would count on my Penn State transcript. I loved being among a group of Black students from HBCUs *and* PWIs—Predominantly White Institutions—from all over the country, all of us striving for a similar goal. As smart and impressive as the Black students from PWIs were, that summer shaped my view of HBCUs: Their students were—are—equally brilliant or more, equally capable of profound ideas, impressive action, inspiring leadership.

In the fall, I transferred to the main Penn State campus, University Park in State College, where there were more activities and way more undergrads than at Penn State-Behrend. All of it was new to me.

I got a work-study job at the Paul Robeson Cultural Center, which housed a library and gym, and hosted lots of parties. I felt such admiration for Robeson, who seemed larger than life. He was a renowned singer, author, activist, humanitarian, athlete, lawyer, actor, scholar. Most of the students who came into the center were Black. My job was simple: Sit at the front desk and check out books. When things were quiet, I studied, while earning slightly more than minimum wage—enough to have money in my pocket but not much more.

I was initiated into Alpha Kappa Alpha Sorority, Incorporated. My sisters were very ladylike; I was tomboyish. That was partly my personality and also because being fly and feminine was expensive. But my sisters loved me for me. They braided my hair. They let me borrow their dressy, cool clothing. Because I was studying so much, I often missed practice for our "step shows," but they were only too eager to teach me the steps after I returned to the dorm. They knew I was all about the books and they celebrated me for it. The sisterhood helped bolster my confidence and embrace womanhood.

And I fell in love with Penn State football, which was something of an anomaly for a Black girl there. As a Lion Ambassador, I worked on "card block," where you coordinate fans in a giant student section to create an image with cards, or spell out a message. Pretty much all the spectators were white. I don't know why more Black students didn't attend the games when so many of us were playing. One possible reason: Games were expensive. Another one: The music was not what we listened to. But there was likely a darker reason, too: There were always white folks in the stadium who'd get drunk and make ignorant racist comments. On several occasions, as I walked back from the stadium, a bunch of drunk white guys called out the n-word from the car.

And there were separate homecomings. Yes, a white homecoming and a Black homecoming. Don't get me wrong: They didn't *advertise* it like that, but that's more or less what happened. That was life at Penn State, at least when I was there.

That winter, home from college for Kwanzaa and Christmas, I told my family that I needed to do well on the MCAT, and to do *that*, I needed to take a Stanley Kaplan prep class, which cost $1,000 (a *lot* of money then). At a holiday gathering, one of the elders started passing a hat and everyone chipped in—some $5, some $10, some $100, some checks, and some coins. By the end of the evening, I had enough for the class.

People are smart in different ways. Some have high emotional intelligence. Some are fast processors. Some have great recall. Some have a great spatial sense. There were lots of things I could do well: Acing standardized tests was not one of them. I did respectably on the MCAT on my first try, good enough that my dream of medical school—any medical school—didn't die then and there.

Why wasn't I better at it? Part of it is just the way I'm wired, I guess. But part of it was that I wasn't educated, at least not until college, in the way that standardized tests reward. How you grow up significantly affects how you think and process. The vocabulary you hear growing up matters. The conversations in your household matter. With a single mom, one who was working all the time and rarely home, I was simply not exposed to some of the words on the test, words they presume you know. Today, when I listen to my teenaged children, they sound to me like grown men. Not because of their tone—they still sound like boys to me—but in their vocabulary. To this day, when I read a book and come across words I don't know, I write them in the back to look up later. I am a perpetual learner.

I didn't think about it at the time, and far fewer people talked about it then, but: Who wrote the test questions? Who came up with the concepts to be tested? We now know that it was predominantly white men educated in a similar way.[1] However objective they strived to be, they couldn't help but be influenced by their background, as we all are. And that particular background, so different from mine and people like me, determined what was being tested and rewarded. Is the MCAT really the best way to find our best doctors? Is the LSAT the best way to weed out the best lawyers? Are standardized tests the best way to find the next generation of best *anything*s? The background of the people formulating the tests did not represent the diversity of the people taking them. Fortunately, there's now lots of literature about this, much of which debunks the correlation between performance on tests and performance out in the world.

After junior year, on June 1, the very first day you could apply to medical school, I was at the post office with all my applications, waiting to have them postmarked. I applied to eight schools, no more, because each application was expensive, around $200—another obvious disadvantage for poorer kids.

I landed several interviews. I could not have been more thrilled, but they did not all go according to plan. At Temple University's medical school, the interviewer looked at my application and said, "Are you sure you don't want to apply to *law* school? You seem more like the activist type, not a physician." That hurt my heart to hear, especially coming from a school in my hometown. I worried I had gone about things all wrong.

Then I waited. Fall of senior year, right before Thanksgiving, it arrived. I will never forget the moment, the feeling. How *can* you forget, when it's the thing you've been dreaming about since you were eight years old?

From Jefferson Medical College in Philadelphia, the embossed letter began:

Ala Stanford,

It is a pleasure to inform you that you have been accepted into the Class of '96 Jefferson Medical College.

As I tell young people who yearn to be doctors: It takes only one med school acceptance.

I got my second acceptance, to Penn State College of Medicine-Hershey, which offered me more financial aid than Jefferson. Temple University School of Medicine sent me a rejection letter.

I chose Penn State not only because of the financial aid, but also because their class size was significantly smaller—a little over 100 students versus 250+ at Jefferson, where I feared I might get lost. True, Jefferson was ranked higher than Penn State-Hershey at the time, but I knew of at least ten people of color going to Penn State—a decent number, especially then, in a class of 100. (That's not to say that Jefferson had no students of color.) Also, Jefferson was in Philly, and I knew I couldn't be there. Too distracting. Whenever I returned home during college, I saw too many people—friends, people from the neighborhood—who were doing nothing with their lives. It wasn't healthy for me. Heather, fresh off her graduation from Hampton University in Virginia, had moved further south to Atlanta, to get her master's in engineering at Georgia Tech.

Thanks to that summer prep program at Harvard, I had enough credits to graduate early from Penn State University with a bachelor's degree in Biology. I was twenty years old. I couldn't even legally have a celebratory drink.

Medical school didn't start until summer, so I looked for a job and landed one, thanks to my Bio degree. I worked as a research assistant at SmithKline Beecham (now GlaxoSmithKline). I enjoyed looking at things under the microscope, growing cultures in Petri dishes, identifying them, checking cell growth, using flasks and micropipettes, taking care not to shake the flask or otherwise mess up the milieu—there's a word I wasn't exposed to growing up—making sure the solution was the right temperature. The project looked at kidney cells and inflammation, both congenital and acquired. It reminded me of how I loved using the magnifying glass on grade school field trips.

Still, it was just a means to an end.

THE SOURCE OF OUR
OWN RIVER

I nearly flunked out of medical school. I also tell *that* to young people yearning to be doctors. It can happen. Don't give up. It's hard. If it were easy, everyone would do it.

It was a challenge for me. The challenge wasn't always about my being Black, or a woman, or a Black woman. But a lot of the time it wasn't *not* about that, either. And sometimes it absolutely *was* about that.

Early in my time at Penn State College of Medicine-Hershey, on a general surgery rotation, one of the attending surgeons asked the half-dozen of us medical students to list the Ranson's criteria, which indicates the level of severity for pancreatitis.* I started to answer when he interrupted me. "Never mind, the girls never know anyway," he said, half-laughing. I proceeded with my answer—and again he stopped me cold. One of the male students chimed in, allowed to finish exactly what I was going to say.

---

*An "attending" doctor is fully credentialed and supervises and teaches medical students, interns, and residents.

That wasn't the only older male surgeon who did not expect us female medical students to go on to become surgeons. And if we weren't (was his thinking), why waste time? Ours or his? Maybe it was a victory that I got to blurt out even a few words. It definitely triggered my "if you want me to do something, tell me I can't" mentality.

As a med student, I didn't see inequitable treatment toward patients as much as I heard about it. In classes and discussions about particular medical histories, the professor or section leader might recount what a patient of meager economic means—very often Black—had done, or likely not done, to contribute to his or her compromised condition. How they had *not* taken control of their health. How they had *not* advocated for themselves. The picture was clear: Somehow their poor health was their fault. Somehow it had nothing to do with their marginalization. Nothing to do with the lack of resources and access to care. Or because past, infamous atrocities throughout the health care system, dangerous and terrible treatments that were exposed only years or decades later, had made Black people justifiably wary of doctors, medications, and procedures, even routine checkups and fairly generic recommendations. Or because there were so few doctors and health care authority figures with brown faces like the people walking through the doors of hospitals and clinics and doctors' offices, seeking someone they could trust. Or because even present-day doctors spend less time, on average, talking with a Black patient, partly because they think the patient won't understand what's being said, can't afford the cost of care, or won't follow the instructions.[1]

The fundamental problem was an untrustworthy health care system, one that had broadly, consistently failed Black Americans.

I was disappointed to hear the built-in biases coming out of the mouths of highly esteemed doctors, but I did not pipe up, not then. I had worked too hard to get where I was, and it didn't seem the time or place to rock the boat. When I began to feel angry and helpless about what was being implied—more than implied—I thought, *I'm going to change this one day.* I had hope because I was going to be a doctor, and doctors are respected authority figures, and then I would be able to make a difference.

I nearly flunked out because with the approach of my first big exam, the one you had to pass or you were done, my head was elsewhere. My mother, my foundation, needed a major operation. (I wanted to donate blood but I was anemic; Kamau came through.) Then one night, as I exited the library after hours of studying, I thought I noticed my brother's car. It was him, Kamau, sitting in the car. "Is that you?" *What on earth?* He looked as if he'd seen a ghost. He told me he'd been pulled over by the Philly cops—profiled, searched, he felt horribly violated—and after they released him he didn't know where to go. So he drove all the way to Hershey, to me. He needed to escape the city, for me to listen and to just be. Days later, the dean very kindly gave me an extension on the exam when I told him how distracted I'd been by my personal life.

When I took the test, I passed, barely. I mean . . . *barely*.

It's tough being a medical student, tougher being a Black one. Or, as one Black mentor said, being a tiny raisin in a big glass of milk. Black students made up one-tenth of our medical school class. There were two Hispanic students and a few Asian Americans, but otherwise it was almost entirely white. There was lots of self-segregating during study time, with most of the Black students sitting together in the library, and the white students huddling, as well.

It wasn't until I occasionally branched out from my core group of Black students that I came to a realization: Certain study materials existed that we weren't privy to. Simple as that. Resources built over years, even generations, of med students—fathers, grandfathers, mothers who had paved the way and gone through all of this before. *Generational knowledge*, kind of like generational wealth. We lacked the pipeline some of the white students had because their parents or older siblings were doctors. They had the benefit of old tests and study guides that we never saw, and the ability to phone a relative or close family friend who was a doctor and only too happy to share their experience, maybe their connections, too. (I had my cousin Christophe, but he was pretty busy himself as an anesthesia resident.) The white students—not all, of course, but not a tiny number, either—had these materials, like a secret stash, and they weren't about to share, because anything that can give you an upper hand in med school, you take. Every so often I would get a glance at the "other" study material, but that was it. Me and my Black classmates? We were starting from scratch. We had to create our own, and maybe it would be a pipeline for our kids someday. We would have to be the source of our own river. Those of us who had started with less, who had fewer (or zero) connections to medical school, were at a clear disadvantage. So I—we—would have to work that much harder.

One man in our group worked hardest of all: While we each liked to think we couldn't be outworked, Malcolm was the true champ. When the last of our group would give in and finally leave the med school library at 1:30 or 2:00 in the morning, Malcolm was still there, cranking. We were back in our dorm rooms sleeping, and he was still at it. Malcolm got the best grades of anyone—white or Black—and it was thrilling and inspiring to see him excelling in everything. It was only later that we found out that when the last of us had quit the library, leaving Malcolm alone, that he was homeless. When he left the library, it was to walk to his car, to sleep.

Today, he's an incredible, highly respected cardiologist doing amazing things.

When I wasn't in libraries I was often in bookstores, mainly Barnes & Noble, getting lost in books. (It's sad that there are so few of them to get lost in today.) Like a moth to a flame, I just about always ended up in one of three sections: African American Authors, Self-Help, or faith books and Bibles. I was almost twenty-two, still in my first year of medical school, when I pulled a book off the shelf titled, *The Courage to Heal: A Guide for Women Survivors of Child Sexual Abuse* by Ellen Bass and Laura Davis.

The book had such profound wisdom to impart. About giving no things power over you. About reaching the point that you stop wrestling with your past. The book quickly became absolutely vital to me, as did the companion workbook, which I carried wherever I went. But I didn't want anyone to see the books in my backpack. I didn't want anyone knowing I was reading them, and didn't want them making judgments about me.

That year I also found time to read Ralph Ellison's novel *Invisible Man*, and felt the spark of recognition. Like the unnamed narrator, I was trying to fit in where they hadn't really set out a place for people like me to fit. I was so impressed by Ellison's courage, talent, and skill. That book, too, would shape me more than I knew.

In some ways, I was very fortunate to be at Penn State-Hershey, because of a man whose job it was to make sure the students of color felt supported. Dr. Alphonse Leure-duPree, born and raised in Haiti, professor of neural and behavioral sciences and associate dean for academic achievement, was a one-man force. He fostered a community among the ten of us. That's why we studied together: because everyone needs community. It helped enormously to get to know a doctor of color so widely renowned and respected. It's crucial to have a mentor who will go to bat for you.

There's not enough of that in the Black medical community, not close to enough. Earlier I wrote that fewer than 6 percent of doctors in the United States are African American. Distressingly, that figure has hardly budged in the last quarter-century. Even more startling, in 1940, Black men represented 2.7 percent of the American physician workforce. In 2018, almost eighty years later? They represented 2.6 percent of the physician workforce.[2] This matters enormously, not just for a future with more Black doctors, but for the physical and mental health and well-being of Black patients right now. Several recent research papers show that many white medical students bring with them to medical school certain biases about Black patients—about their health outcomes, and why those outcomes are as poor as they often are. And these biases, so often, are simply wrong. These supposedly objective, scientific assessments are rooted in biased misinformation, yet the students come into medical school unaware of that. These biases can be addressed and overcome, but to do so takes work and a willingness to acknowledge the cracks in the system. It's one big reason why we need more doctors of color. We all have preconceived notions about things. But if the next generation of doctors is dominated by people unfamiliar with *why* certain health disparities are the way they are, then we're guaranteeing more years of suboptimal care and choices. The majority of white medical practitioners do a very good job at what they do, but if the culture teaches or influences them in a certain misguided way about Black health, it's no wonder we still have unusually poor outcomes. Evidence has shown that having even one Black doctor on staff improves cultural competence and patient outcomes—just one![3]

Then there are the expectations and unfounded notions of the medical school staff and faculty. It felt as if virtually all the Black and Latino students were being pushed to go into primary care. This pressure was prevalent at my school, but it's a phenomenon still observed at medical schools all over the country. Sometimes it was an explicit exhortation—*We need doctors to go into communities and take care of the underserved! Aren't those your people?* Sometimes it was more implicit. Med school students are often recruited to take part in community service projects. Guess which students are predominantly the ones who engage in these activities at elementary schools, high schools, churches, shelters, wherever? Doing frog and heart dissections and the like? (Don't get me wrong: I enjoyed my time participating in these. As a schoolkid, I would have *loved* for a young med student to show me the various chambers of the heart.) The problem is that many of those medical students of color are exactly the ones who need to be in class more, not less, and they're not. Serve your own—and fall behind? Or study—and turn your back on your own?

If a young doctor goes into primary care, they might have their medical school debt erased, which is huge for anyone, but particularly for individuals who don't come from generational wealth. That's good, right? Yes, it's very, very good. But it also means that for the rest of your medical career, the goal that you trained so hard to reach, you are compensated at a far lower level than practitioners in other disciplines.

Pressure and guilt didn't work on me. Tell me I have to do something or should do something and you've pretty much guaranteed I won't. In fact, I entered medical school thinking that I *wanted* to return to my community and help folks. I was aware that my community and ones like it were among those in greatest need of help. And if that wasn't reason enough, then yeah, sure, I would have loved starting my post–medical school career debt-free. Very tempting.

But the more I felt the pressure, the more I resisted. I didn't just resent being pushed to go into primary care, or that it was less well-paying than many other fields, and less well-respected. It was also that primary care or family medicine doctors practice in run-down facilities with inferior equipment. I wasn't the only young Black doctor who thought, *Oh, so basically you want to ship me back to where I came from, right? Somehow it's my job as a Black doctor, a Black woman doctor, to fix this broken system? In broken buildings, with second-rate equipment?*

When I had those thoughts, I recoiled. I wanted to make my own choice. I worked so hard to get to medical school. And there was so much work ahead of me. After med school, I would spend years training in my chosen area before I would be eligible to sit for my boards, then there'd be *more* years of training if I wanted to go into a specialty, before I could sit for *those* boards. There might be more years—research perhaps—tacked on.

Yes, I wanted to be there for the neighborhood and the city that raised me. In fact, I had promised myself that I would do something specifically for my home community, someday, somehow. How could I not? I was one of the lucky ones. Kamau was one of the lucky ones.

But right now, this was *my* dream, *my* life, *my* world. No one but me was going to dictate the direction.

· · ·

My second year in med school we did our psychiatry block, learning relevant skills like how to interview someone with mental health challenges. Now it was time to put what we'd studied into action. We convened in a large, banked amphitheater. Smiling and eager, I sat as always, in the front row. A man, a patient with an actual problem—not an actor—entered, along with our professor, who did not tell us the man's diagnosis, just that it was a condition in the *Diagnostic and Statistical Manual of Mental Disorders, Fourth Edition*—better known as *DSM-IV*. It would be up to one of us to figure out his condition.

The professor asked for a student to volunteer to come up and interview the patient. Naturally, I raised my hand.

We couldn't outright ask the classroom visitor, "Are you schizophrenic?" or "Do you suffer from depression?" That's not how therapy, or at least good therapy, is done. We had to come to the answer by deduction and induction, asking questions like, "What's your home situation?" Maybe he would answer that he was living in a halfway house, or that he'd just been released from prison. From there, we could build on information we were methodically gathering. I strode down, front and center, and took a seat maybe three feet from the man.

"Hello, I'm glad you're here today," I said, trying to make him feel comfortable. "I'm glad you decided to talk to someone, so you can feel better about you." I paused, waiting for a response. He did not look ready to talk. "Would you like to share with me?"

Everything that happened next is hazy.

He began talking about urges. He said something disjointed about how the child seemed as if they wanted to be part of whatever it was he was trying to do. I remember him saying he felt remorse. That he recognized that it was wrong.

I had entered a fugue state. It felt as if it took everything in my power to maintain my composure, not to break down in tears.

I couldn't ask, "Are you a child molester?" But that's exactly what he was.

My whole class, approximately one hundred med students, was silent in the amphitheater, as they observed our back-and-forth, listening to this man talk about molesting children, with me sitting just a few feet away trying to act as a cool, unfazed clinician.

In a brief moment of clarity, I felt anger at my professor, who *knew* that the interviewee was an actual former (or current!) child molester. But that feeling passed. It wasn't the professor's fault. He didn't know *my* history.

I kept asking the man questions, being the dutiful med student. (At least I think I did.) But the only thing that echoed in my brain were his words, *I thought they wanted it.*

I held it together, somehow. I did not cry. When it was over, as I returned from the stage to my front-row seat, I remember my professor saying, "Nice job, Ala." There may have been applause from my classmates. Then *blah, blah, blah.*

I managed to slip out of the amphitheater, probably wearing a forced smile.

Back in my apartment, I had to clean myself. My boyfriend came over and entered the bathroom while I was in the shower—I freaked out. When I finally caught my breath, I explained to him what had happened in class. He was sympathetic—at first. "God, that's horrible . . . horrible," he cooed. But then he touched me, and I recoiled. He was surprised and no doubt hurt by my reaction.

"*I* didn't do it to you," he said.

I couldn't believe his response.

I went into a tailspin after that. Spiraling, spinning. Everything bubbled up. I had just participated in a real-life Q&A diagnosis for our psychiatry block in med school . . . and now *I* was the one having a psychological breakdown. Or PTSD. Call it what you will. I couldn't function. I didn't leave my room for days. I wasn't ready to deal with "it" or anyone. I felt as if I had no one to talk to.

Heather was at Georgia Tech, head down, studying engineering. I couldn't talk to my mom about it: Those assholes who had abused me, those motherfuckers, were men she had invited into our home. Of course, she didn't know they would hurt her child. And if I *did* try to talk to her, *with* her, I knew I would have to go through all of her drama first about how she hadn't known, not for a long time, and then all that she'd had to endure herself, and all this other shit, none of which would be helpful to me. Yes, she had me when she was fourteen, and she was thrown out of the house for getting pregnant. She had Kamau when she was nineteen. And she was a single mom, working all the time and doing the best she could with what she had. I got all that—I got it, I got it, okay?—I absorbed it all a long time ago. But if she thought she was helping when she told me, so defensively, back when I was in high school, "It doesn't matter who you tell, because I've already told every-one, and there's no point in you asking Grandma if she recalls this or that because they already know. They know that this is just something that happened" . . . yeah, that really didn't help, either.

I couldn't call my father because he didn't know the extent of what had happened in the past, and he would have felt horrible again, more so, guilty that he wasn't there for me and should have been. There was a time, about the end of middle school, where I was sure he had to have an inkling about the first one and maybe the beginning of the second, and I was screaming inside, *Why didn't anyone warn me about this? Why didn't you, Daddy?* Because *that's what he did for a living! Investigate child abuse and keep predators away from children!* I must have been trying so hard to have him always see us in a good light and not make my mom look bad. Because that would mean just one more time that Kamau and I wouldn't get to spend with him, that he wouldn't pick us up.

Lying there in my bed in my apartment in Hershey, PA, curled up, staring at the ceiling, I knew one thing: I couldn't fall apart. I couldn't allow it. I was going to be a doctor, no matter what. That didn't waver. But part of me now felt trapped.

Being up close, "interviewing" an abuser who was doing his best to justify for me and the whole class of medical students why his ac-tions were okay . . . how could I not collapse? Everything I had tried to suppress from my childhood, that I had tried to move on from—it was all right there in my face.

I talked with my boyfriend, but he had only so much patience for what I was saying or what I needed. I realized I was done with him, which hurt because he had been one of my few sanctuaries of support in the combat zone known as medical school. I thought of calling Claudette, my friend from Lockport and the one I'd told more of this stuff to than anyone, more even than Heather.

Instead, I called the hospital ER. "I need to come in because I'm concerned I could hurt myself," I told them.

I was admitted. There, at least, I felt safe. I talked to a psychiatrist. I was able to sleep. My second day there, walking around the unit, I saw all sorts of damaged folks. I looked at them like the medical student I was: trying to identify the pathology all around me. Nurses brought them medication. During one of my hour-long sessions with the therapist, I said of my fellow patients, "These folks are broken, really broken. Maybe they don't even know they're broken. They're not capable of knowing. And that's part of the problem." I paused. "This is not what I thought it was going to be like."

"What did you think it would be like?" the therapist asked.

"I thought I would talk to someone and get through all this and . . . whatever. This isn't what I thought. I want to leave."

They would allow it as long as I committed to therapy twice per week, and started medication for depression, Zoloft. I agreed to the conditions.

It was one of the best things I ever did. It started me on a long, slow path to healing. I didn't want what happened to me when I was a child to dictate the rest of my life.

I had to pick my specialty. Yeah, you guessed right: Psychiatry would *not* be it.

It wasn't just the horrible experience with the child molester in the amphitheater. As a discipline it wasn't the right energy for me. As most doctors know, no matter the medical field you go into—dentistry, podiatry, orthopedics—your patient will tell you how he or she is feeling, physically, mentally. And that's not a bad thing; don't get me wrong. But I didn't want to make that the focus of my day. Psychiatry was knocked off the list.

Radiology was also a no. I'm someone who needs bright light, so sitting in a dark room all day looking at X-rays and scans would have depressed me. The one thing that *did* appeal to me about radiology? No scrubs. I could wear nice clothes.

Pathology—the study of disease—while interesting, was smelly, plus I didn't like being around so much dead tissue and tumors. One way or the other, nearly every doctor deals with pathology, at least its conclusions. I didn't mind examining cadavers in my Harvard Medical School summer program but I didn't need examples of it in my face every day.

Internal medicine? It meant you talked and talked and talked all day. As it was generally practiced, everything was presumed to be curable with medicine and only medicine. Oh, that medicine doesn't work? No problem, try this one. I'm not anti-medicine, but I felt as if there wasn't enough support for nonmedicine therapies and lifestyle changes. I imagined that, for me, internal medicine would feel like watching paint dry.

Obstetrics seemed cool. I was confident I would be good at it. Childbirth is the most beautiful thing in the world to witness. The miracle of it made me feel my faith in God, same as when I watch a sunrise or sunset. And obstetrics was fun—all those babies! The deliveries were fun. But there, too, obstetrics didn't quite fit my personality. Maybe a little too much estrogen for me. When you choose a specialty, you're also choosing the people you'll be working with, so you want to find a sense of camaraderie, and I wasn't feeling that with obstetrics.

I loved pediatrics but it didn't challenge me enough. I saw so much of myself in the kids. I could be with them all day. They brightened everything. As much as I was there for them, they were there for me. But I needed to be selfish, to do what I wanted, because this was my life, my formative years.

At the time, I didn't know that pediatric surgery was so lucrative; I did know that it was one of the most competitive, coveted fields. I knew that surgery challenged me, and that children made me happy. The combination seemed perfect. *Gifted Hands*, the book by Dr. Ben Carson, had made an impact on me: Someone who looked like me, from a background like mine, had become a renowned doctor, changing children's lives for the better, forever. Add to that the great respect that pediatric surgeons, as I gradually came to see, earned from even their surgical colleagues. It was like, *Oh, my gosh, she's a pediatric surgeon! She's smart!* Pediatric surgeons have to know everything that general surgeons know—and more. Before they let you operate on a child, you have to perfect your technique on adults. The volume of blood in a newborn is about that of a can of soda. Their body cavity is so small, you often can't see what you're doing. Touch an organ wrong and you may do irreparable harm.

The discipline also offered me a certain, very personal level of healing: I got to protect these children when they were in my presence, and my responsibility. I was their advocate, which allowed me in some ways to heal for myself, because I felt as if I hadn't had my own protector as a child.

And then there's the art and technique of surgery. Intellectually, it stimulated me. It challenged me. It required me to study harder; it made me *want* to study harder. I simply couldn't get enough of it. Learning new procedures excited me. In the OR, when I was on the anesthesia rotation, standing behind the curtain, I so badly wanted to be right there in the center of the action, standing over the patient, performing the operation. Yes, it's a performance. As I listened to the anesthesiologist teaching us about gasses and ventilators, my head and

heart were elsewhere, on the other side of the drape, cutting and su-
turing. I wanted to understand it more. And technically, I was good
at it.

Everything about surgery felt exciting. To me, everything else in
medicine and health care was easy by comparison.

6

IF YOU'RE NOT IN THE HOSPITAL, YOU'D BETTER BE IN THE HOSPITAL

Every doctor can tell you about the hardships of medical education and training. The years drag on, the academics are demanding, the work is hard, sometimes it feels as if you haven't slept for months. You need every bit of drive to keep at it. Medical school is medical school.

But post–medical school—internship (the first year of residency) and the rest of residency, where you're training full-time—is even harder. The work. The hours. The pressure. Those who strive to make it harder for you. Knowing you'll either make it or you won't, with no real in-between. Learning from your mistakes and the errors of others. The difficulty of sustaining relationships. The possibility of endangering a life even as you're trying to save it. The sacrifices that come with success are brutal for almost anyone who goes through it. But in the years—and years—between medical school and becoming an attending surgeon, I also had to face racism and sexism, sometimes subtle, sometimes blatant.

On that day in March when all med school grads open their envelopes to see where they've "matched" (you rank your preferred institutions, they rank their preferred candidates), I got State University of New York-Downstate, in Kings County—better known as Brooklyn.

Brooklyn was a mixed bag. One positive: It was incredibly diverse. Sometimes I felt like I was the minority—but not because I was a minority in America, or part of an underrepresented group in a particular environment. No, I mean I was *in* the minority—but then, so was everyone else, because there were people from so many places and backgrounds. Russian folks, Jewish folks, Arab folks, Caribbean, African, Indian, Asian, Hispanic. So many sub-groups within those larger ones. We felt like we were all in it together.

The work and hours were brutal. After work there was usually time to eat, sleep, or wash your body, but not all three in a night. As surgeons in training, we were so busy at the hospital, rounding on our patients, writing orders and notes, changing dressings, debriding wounds, placing central lines, assisting in the operating room (if you were lucky), then soon enough doing the operations ourselves. Once the attending surgeons felt we had a particular procedure down, we were more or less on our own. *See one, do one, teach one.* But they made you earn it; I was never quite sure if they were trying to teach me or break me.

Once, as an intern, I was assisting the surgeon in the OR on a vascular anastomosis for a dialysis graft, a procedure that required meticulous moves and extremely fine suture. We were seated, our face masks not ten inches from each other.

"Why would you choose something so difficult as surgery?" he asked. "When you could have chosen medicine or pediatrics, something less demanding?" Similar queries continued the remainder of the operation, as I placed every stitch, tied every knot, even as I cut suture. *You're not good enough and you don't belong here.* I held back the tears as best I could, but I was failing. My mask grew damp. My glasses fogged until I almost couldn't see.

I got mad. I deserved to be there. I was angry at myself for allowing him to see me cry and that he was the reason why. I cleaned myself up at the scrub sink and in that moment decided never again to let him—or anyone like him—bring me to tears.

All of us got very, very good at what we did. Unfortunately, we saw lots of wounds from gun violence and injuries from child abuse.

There were nine of us young surgeons, all between the ages of twenty-five and twenty-seven. You bond with work colleagues, but even more so when everyone's going through the same crap. For instance, we all had to do our own blood draws on patients. The nurses didn't do it and there was no dedicated phlebotomy team; county hospitals like ours tended to be understaffed. At five in the morning, often earlier, for every patient on our rounds we drew blood, took the tubes down to the lab, and got a printout of results for when rounds started at six and our chief resident inevitably asked for the info. Same with X-rays: It was on us to have them in hand (though not actually to take them) in their paper jacket. (This was before digital images.)

My peers and I worked well and fast—we *had* to work fast. I was one of the youngest doctors in that group. As the saying went, "There are no men and no women, just surgeons," and it felt like that—among my peers (if not always my superiors), I didn't feel judged.

But being a young Black woman doctor among so many young Black women nurses, I felt something new: resentment. *Why should I respect you?* was the vibe I got from them. *You're the same age as me. You have an MD and I have an RN—that doesn't make you better than me, honey. You certainly don't work harder than me.*

It wasn't all of them, of course. Many of the older nurses looked out for me. Perhaps the ones around my age were more competitive, had more of a chip on their shoulder. We were all strugglin' to survive.

I let all the nurses know how much I valued them. How I couldn't do my job without them. How much they could teach me because they'd been doing this way longer. Earning their respect took work.

My training was in general surgery, but just about every month we focused on a different surgical subspecialty: thoracic, critical care, pediatric, transplant, vascular, oncology, etc. I did my first laparoscopic procedure, using four little strawlike instruments to perform a cholecystectomy, the removal of the gallbladder. I attached a photo of the gallbladder on my boyfriend's refrigerator with a magnet. Then I did a laparoscopic appendectomy. I was learning fast.

As young, constantly working surgeons at Kings County, we gained a reputation as people who could save your life, but *not* for being book-smart. Far from it. Each year we had to take an "in-service" exam, which supposedly predicted our aptitude for passing the general surgery boards a few years down the road. Basically: Did we absorb the material they'd been teaching us? Did we have command of the knowledge to someday be a chief resident? With all the surgery and follow-up patient care, there wasn't much time for studying. As in, none.

The first year at Kings County, most of our scores were in the single-digit percentiles—6th percentile (meaning 94 percent of test-takers did better), 11th, etc. Like, astoundingly horrible. If one of us got, say, a 38th percentile—still not remotely a great score—we celebrated. A program director posted all of our pathetic in-service scores on their office door, inside the glass, so it could not be removed. All the nurses, other residents, and basically anyone walking past that office could see how badly we'd done; could see that if we hotshot young surgeons ever portrayed ourselves as being all that, here was proof that we were actually pretty dumb. (Can you imagine a superior doing that today? Neither can I.)

Why did we still have jobs as surgeons despite our poor test scores? Because we were good surgeons. In-service exams don't test hand-eye coordination, for example, or resourcefulness, or bedside manner. Who could fault us for being bad test-takers when we were routinely working entire days and nights, and 100+ hour workweeks? On my drives home after being on call basically for thirty-six consecutive hours, I got into the habit of shifting my car into park at red lights: There was a high likelihood that I would fall asleep at the wheel, and I didn't want to awaken (or not awaken) to find that my car had rolled into the intersection. It happened more than once.

For some of my colleagues, it was all too much. They quit, including several of my Black peers.

Or worse. One morning, a surgical intern a year younger did not show up at work. You were never late for rounds. Never. Our chief resident, who knew many of the local police by name, got a cop to drive to the intern's home to check on him. He had hanged himself.

The news spread quickly, but the tragedy wasn't formally acknowledged until our weekly morbidity and mortality conference, held in the auditorium, when one of the attending surgeons took his turn at the podium and announced, "We had a loss." He said another sentence or two—I don't remember what—then asked for a moment of silence, which lasted ten seconds, tops. And that was that. On to the business at hand. We were expected to proceed as if nothing had happened. Back then there was no "If you need to talk to someone about it, we have counselors." Some of us sat in the auditorium, crying. It didn't matter.

A few days later, we interns were given the afternoon off to attend our colleague's funeral. I didn't realize until then that he had an identical twin brother. The brother, in full Navy regalia, stood stone-still guard over his brother's open casket, a body that looked exactly like him. Afterward, we hugged his family, then all of us interns and second years—stunned, but maybe not as stunned as we ought to have been—took over a bar in Manhattan and drank all night. At 4:30 in the morning, it was time to go to work again.

There's something very wrong there.

Such cold pragmatism was not uncommon. It almost seemed as if at least one trainee, from across all the Kings County programs, committed suicide just about every year. The mantra for residency, especially the most intense ones (surgery, anesthesia, obstetrics), was simple: If you're not in the hospital, you'd better be *in* the hospital. That is, there was no acceptable excuse for not being present and contributing unless you were laid up in a hospital bed. Every now and then, one of us would be found dead, maybe overdosed in a hospital closet, having injected propofol or fentanyl between our toes. Sick and sad as it is to admit this, on those incredibly rare instances when someone had the nerve to fail to appear for their shift, we simply assumed suicide. And kept working.

What troubled me and so many others was not just the horror of a young doctor believing that suicide was the most rational way out of their situation. It was also the psychological climate, the *reaction* to such a wrenching emotional event by seasoned medical people, who had supposedly become doctors at least partly out of an impulse to care for people. Later in my training, a friend and surgical resident at a Boston hospital suffered a miscarriage. She was on call and explained to her superior the loss she had suffered. "I know I'm supposed to take call tonight, but I can't," she said. Her supervisor, the chief resident, looked at her, uncomprehending. "The baby's already dead," he said. She finished her call shift and quit the next day.

"Trauma" was the byword for those we treated and also for ourselves. One night, we received a patient who had been hit by a subway train. Everything about him looked disfigured beyond recognition, but he was able to communicate enough to say, "Don't let me die." He was a tourist, we learned, and he'd been pushed onto the tracks, though whether it was intentional or accidental we didn't know, and that fact was irrelevant at the moment. He died in the trauma bay, before we could get him to the OR.

Then there were the homeless patients who lived in our hospital's stairwell. We used the stairs constantly because the elevators were commandeered by clinical staff moving patients in gurneys—that is, when the old elevators weren't broken. For most of us young doctors, it was just faster to take the stairs. And when the New York weather turned cold, we noticed a person or two had set up camp in the ground level of the stairwell to get warm. *Don't mess with them, they won't mess with you*, was the understanding. *Just keep moving.*

We had a patient who lived in the hospital. After being treated and officially released, he simply refused to leave. We couldn't kick him out: If you say you have a medical condition (his was diverticulitis; he had just undergone a colostomy) and that you have nowhere to go (he said he had no room or even mattress), you can't be moved. Within weeks he was giving the hospital as his address and started receiving mail there. Finally, someone at the hospital found a halfway house for him. To help ease the patient's transition, Roger, one of our chief residents, bought a mattress with his own money. "If he has a new mattress, he'll leave," Roger figured. He tied it to the roof of his car and chauffeured our hospital dweller to his new home.

As young surgeons we didn't just rotate through different specialties with different attending surgeons, we also rotated through different hospitals. I did time at Long Island College Hospital in Brooklyn, St. Vincent's Hospital in Staten Island, and Lenox Hill Hospital in Manhattan, which had a NICU to manage premature infants. There was no staff pediatric surgeon in house there, but emergencies inevitably arose, and before I knew it, I became the surgeon who handled them: See one, do one, teach one.

Put a drain in this baby that weighs half a pound?

Guess what, Ala? It's your turn.

Damn. Okay. A preemie was suffering from a pneumoperitoneum—air or gas in the abdomen, often caused by a perforated bowel or intestine—and I aspirated the abdomen with a needle to decompress it. This allowed the infant to take deeper breaths. Prior to my intervention, the baby's abdomen was taut and shiny like a rubber ball filled with water. Then I made a cut to insert a Penrose drain (a rubber band tube) to siphon out air and stool. As I removed my hands from placing the drain and secured it, I thought, *Well, I sure hope I did that right.*

(I had.)

For all the camaraderie and intensity at work, I was often lonely outside the hospital. It felt like a more profound loneliness because it was New York City, with millions of people everywhere, all the time. I'd be walking down the street, or riding the subway, among so many strangers, and thinking, *None of these people knows me. Not one is my person.*

I could call home, and sometimes it helped. Heather was in Chicago, after graduating with a master's from Georgia Tech. She was always happy to talk, but she was busier even than I. She and her husband both worked at Xerox. They were building a house. They'd bought a Mercedes and a BMW. Heather was pregnant.

For a while I dated a New York City cop named Shaun, who came from a family of cops. I hadn't expected that, and it helped me gain a better understanding of and respect for police officers. He was a breath of fresh air: When we were together, we could forget about the chaos of our respective professions. With our schedules, though, it was just too difficult to see each other much.

When I could, I'd go to Uncle Frank's church, for services or an incredible hot meal, where they would lay food out in front of me like I was a queen.

When things got especially trying at the hospital, I sometimes called home, often at two or three in the morning. Maybe a patient had died, or I'd seen one too many wounded teens come in, or exhaustion beyond imagining had finally overwhelmed me. Sometimes I spoke with Peter, my mother's husband. They'd married a few years earlier, and he was considerably older. He was a tool-and-die maker at Chrysler from the South Side of Chicago, and he offered a particular type of straightshooter guidance. "Did you do everything you could?" he would ask. "Did you do your best? Did you comfort the family?" I would murmur something, and he would say, "Then hold your head up. You can't save everyone, La." And he would chuckle and tell me he was proud of me.

If I got my mother, she would give me her own brand of tough love, which often worked just as well. "Excuse me?" she would say, if I lamented that a patient of mine had passed. "Did you change your name from Ala to God? You ain't nobody. His will is beyond your will. You're just the middleman. You're just His hands. And if you're His hands and you make the right moves, you ain't got shit to do with what happens." She was right. At a certain point, it was out of my hands.

One night, so exhausted from work and stress, I got in my car but had no clue how I got home safely. I'm sure I fell asleep at the wheel.

Thank you, Jesus.

Tough as it was, we were all in the same boat, us young Brooklyn surgeons. I felt supported. I was learning a lot. And I had found my real love, pediatric surgery. I discovered I loved it during my second rotation. There was nothing else I wanted to do. There was nothing about it that I found boring. Something in these little children was broken, and with my hands I could fix it.

When I was on call overnight I slept in an empty patient room on the pediatric ward. The nurses grew to love me for that; if they needed me, they didn't have to page me. They just walked down the hall. But I did it out of the responsibility I felt for my young patients. In that hospital in that part of Brooklyn, as was (and is) the case in many hospitals in poor and working-class neighborhoods, parents often left their ill children alone at the hospital because they had to work or be home to care for their other kids. Not only did we operate on their children, we baby-sat them, too. The kids spent way too much time in their rooms by themselves, with nobody there to visit or comfort them. I was their surgeon, but I also felt like their guardian and sometimes playmate. With the kids, at least there was no whining and demand-making, as there so often is with adults. Once I operated on a child and made them better, they got to flourish and go back to being a kid.

But there was one big problem for me as a Kings County trainee who wanted someday to be a board-certified pediatric surgeon: At the time, no one from there had ever gone on to match in a pediatric surgery fellowship program. There were only twenty-five spots per year in pediatric surgery programs across the whole country, making it the most competitive surgical subspecialty. (Today, there are approximately fifty programs.) You had to be the cream of the cream of the cream of the crop, and every possible advantage helped—like being affiliated with an institution that had a track record of placing residents in pediatric surgery programs. I could come *back* to Brooklyn to practice as a pediatric surgeon, but I would almost certainly have to go elsewhere to be considered for one of those premier training spots.

During my first year in Brooklyn, I had a full month off. I was advised—no, ordered—to take a vacation. I decided to use the time to drive across the country and think about the best way to pursue my goal. I got as far as Texarkana, a place I'd never heard of, before I gave up, exhausted from the drive but really from the insane pace of my life as a surgeon in the heart of Brooklyn. I dropped off my rental car and planned to return home by bus. There was still plenty of time before I had to be back at work, so I made a big detour to Chicago, which was hosting the annual gathering of the American College of Surgeons, the governing body for surgeons in the U.S. and probably the largest and most important surgical association in the world. I attended a talk by a brilliant transplant surgeon named Dr. Sherilyn Gordon-Burroughs, a Black woman, and the smartest person I had ever heard speak in all my years on this planet. She used all these scientific terms—nitric oxide, dendritic cells, apoptosis, proliferation, flow cytometry. It was basic science and immunology but, damn, did she sound smart. She was dressed impeccably. She commanded the room. After her presentation, she was barraged with questions. She had all the answers.

My God, who are you?

I ran up to her afterward. "Hi, I'm Ala . . . How did you learn to do that? To talk like that?"

"Dr. Henri Ford," she said. She told me that her mentor, the principal investigator in the research lab where she had worked at the University of Pittsburgh Medical Center (UPMC), had taught her so many important things—attention to detail; knowing all the literature on a topic and quoting other people's work, especially if they'll be in your session; succinct responses to questions from the public after your presentation. I knew that Pitt had an excellent record of matching with pediatric programs. And I learned that many surgeons at some point in their young careers had done research, so it was hardly a step backward.

"I want to be like you," I informed her.[*]

I learned that Dr. Ford was attending the conference, too, so I tracked him down. "Dr. Ford, I'm Ala Stanford and I want to be a pediatric surgeon."

He considered me. "What year are you?" he asked.

"Intern."

"So you've been a doctor for, what, three months?"

"Little longer," I acknowledged. "But I know what I want."

"If you still want to do it a year from now, call me."

The rest of the conference, I took in every meeting I could. Dressed in my one nice suit, I sat in the back of the auditorium, listened, and madly took notes.

My second year in Brooklyn I shared my wish to become a pediatric surgeon with an important attending surgeon in the department, a terrible man. He took a puff of his cigarette. We were not supposed to smoke anywhere. He smoked everywhere.

I delivered my news, standing in my scrubs and white coat, and he moved forward, reached inside my open coat, and put his hands on my waist and squeezed.

"Let me see if you have what it takes to become a pediatric surgeon," he said.

After a moment he let go.

And I let it go, though I was thoroughly disgusted.

I next shared my wish to be a pediatric surgeon with Dr. Francisca Velcek, one of the senior surgeons at Kings County, who had always

---

[*]In 2017, almost two decades after that conversation, Sherilyn Gordon-Burroughs was murdered by her husband, who then took his own life.

been supportive. I mentioned that I had met Dr. Henri Ford the summer before.

"He's really good," she said, "and if he wants you in his lab, you'll be in his lab. Call him."

I called Dr. Ford and reintroduced myself. "Last year at the ACS conference in Chicago you told me to call you in a year if I was still serious about pediatric surgery. Well, I'm still serious. I really want this. What do I need to do?"

He told me he was open to having me join him at Pittsburgh, but that I couldn't come without a funding source. We would have to apply for a grant. He already had one from the National Institutes of Health (NIH), so we could apply for a supplemental training grant to pay for me. I wrote a draft, FedExed it to him, and he made changes. Then he FedExed it back to me. We repeated this process—how twentieth-century, right?—until it was ready for submission. When Dr. Ford called to tell me that the grant had been accepted, I was over the moon. I couldn't wait to share the news with my folks and a program director. Their response?

"That's great. Downstate can't pay you to do research at another program."

"That's okay," I said proudly. "I have my own funding. I got a grant!" I had thought of everything, hadn't I?

"Well, when you're down there, I won't guarantee you a spot to complete your general surgery training here."

That was not what I was expecting to hear. I *hadn't* thought of everything. I would be giving up an almost sure thing as a *general* surgeon for the possibility of becoming a special kind of surgeon.

I was wobbly. When I spoke to Dr. Ford, he said, "Ala, I can give you an environment where you can flourish. Where you can be nurtured. Only you know if you have the aptitude to succeed, and sometimes you have to step out on faith."

He was right. Of *course* I was going to step out on faith!

Weirdly, I was not overly concerned about giving up a categorical, secure, and valued position—three more years of general surgery training from Downstate—for a highly speculative opportunity to be a pediatric surgeon; really, an opportunity for an opportunity. I was leaving Brooklyn for Pittsburgh. I thought of what Dr. Ford had said to me. What Sherilyn Gordon-Burroughs had said to me about him and her experience in his lab. Everyone, I would learn, liked and respected Dr. Ford. I didn't have a husband or kids. It was fine for me to be selfish by investing in myself. Time to take a chance on me.

Anyway, did I want to stay in Brooklyn with the misogynistic old chain-smoker putting his hands on me?

When my fellow residents heard I was leaving, they thought I was crazy. "How do you give up a guaranteed spot for something so uncertain?" one asked me. "You don't know if it's going to turn into something. Or if you'll get into another surgery program *ever*."

"Yeah, but I know if I stay, the chances of my becoming a pediatric surgeon are just about zero."

I let a program director know I was leaving. I requested from them a letter stating that I was a general surgery resident leaving in "good standing" who had successfully completed her second year of training.

Whenever I recount that part of my professional journey to people in medicine, they're shocked. How could you know, they ask, how could you leave? Maybe it was best I didn't know. Maybe that's the advantage of being twenty-eight. I packed my stuff into a U-Haul and headed to Pittsburgh.

7

SICK OF THIS

Leaving Brooklyn and the diversity of New York for Pittsburgh was another culture shock. Brooklyn had been a rainbow mix of people. Pittsburgh was anything but. I went from being one of many people of color to one of very few, and as a Black woman I stood out even more. There was one Black woman surgeon, quite a bit older than me. There were two Black women who worked in the lab, neither of them med school graduates. My mentor, Dr. Ford, the surgical fellow, Dr. Jeffrey Upperman, and an attending surgeon, Dr. Edward Barksdale, were also Black, but that was about it. I didn't feel as if I had peers. I often felt like a foreigner because I was treated that way, as if someone had simply handed me this spot while the others there had "earned" everything, at every step, coming from Ivy League schools and A-list programs; and me from Penn State and a mid-tier surgical program at Downstate.[*]

I worked hard. My research papers would ultimately be published

*According to most U.S. rankings then, UPMC was in the Top 20 of general surgery programs to train; SUNY-Downstate was not.

and presented. Among my year, I was the most prolific—but it didn't give me a leg up. I was still an interloper. That was a word I didn't know yet either, but I figured it out soon enough.

I was lucky to have someone in the program to vouch for me, a brilliant staff surgeon whose own career was skyrocketing. Dr. Ford was a bright star, and everybody wanted to be close to him, if only to be in his reflected glory. He didn't embrace me immediately. He showed me tough love. To say he was spare with praise is an understatement. In fact, he told me more than once that there were people in our department who asked him why he was wasting his time on me. I'm not sure which was worse: that they said that to him or that he repeated it to me. Either way, he was going to make me earn my spot. I would have to show him I could do the work. Over and over. And over and over. I had to prove it to him and all the doubters.

I don't want to portray the distanced, often chilly reception I got from others as something completely connected to my race or gender. I was rough around the edges. I was passionate and sometimes righteous. I was not stoic. But a handful of the white women working there treated me as if I didn't belong, plain and simple. Dr. Ford kept telling me: "Just keep your head down and do the work. Let the work speak for itself." But that's hard to do when your supposed comrades, to say nothing of your superiors, say nasty things, either to your face or behind your back. One doctor made no bones about the fact that he thought I didn't belong and didn't want me to succeed. Were they all expressing resentment? Hate? Racism? Sexism? One white female surgeon dissed me to the lone Black female transplant surgeon, not realizing that she and I spoke regularly. The white woman's critique? There was something pathologically wrong with me because "no one should be that happy all the time." My upbeat demeanor, which was authentically me (though I was hardly always happy), and which no doubt made for a good bedside manner, was now a fault. New friends shared what was said about me by those who were anything but friends.

She's not going to smile her way out of this.

She acts jovial because she's really stupid.

She doesn't know anything.

She doesn't deserve to be in the program.

Where'd they find her?

The scorn wasn't the kind of thing I felt now and then. I felt it every single day. To play a game and win the game, you need to know the rules—all of them. And I didn't, not yet. Dr. Ford probably did, but he couldn't teach me everything he knew because he was busy, leading a world-famous lab, surviving himself.

The medical people surrounding me were undeniably brilliant—but unlike my colleagues in Brooklyn, the young surgeons here were all book-smart, incredibly so. They probably killed it on their in-service scores. On the other hand, it was said that "they couldn't operate their way out of a paper bag." Being around them, I felt I had better step up my studying, so I could become a book-smarter person than I was.

The first year in the lab I kept my head down, as instructed. I practically lived in the lab. Why not? I had made a couple of friends between the hospital and the lab—a young man named Ben, a surgical fellow, became a trusted friend—but I hardly knew anyone in Pittsburgh. It helped that great things were happening in our lab. I researched necrotizing enterocolitis in nitric oxide: how nitric oxide could either be damaging or potentially helpful to saving premature children that developed ischemic bowel. I studied the evidence-based literature on the subject. I wrote clinical case reports. Our work got accepted for presentation at national conferences, then published. A hypothesis we created in our lab would eventually be transformed into clinical applications used on patients. "Benchside to bedside"—directly translating lab results into ways to treat actual patients—is the goal of translational (applied) research, and we were doing that. If, back when I was a kid, you had "Ala Stanford will one day be lead author on a research paper titled *Nitric Oxide (NO) Induces Dendritic Cell Apoptosis by Modulating Mitochondrial Membrane Potential and Caspase-3 Activity*" on your Bingo card: Props to you.

That first year at Pitt, Dr. Ford told me he didn't want me just in the lab. He also wanted me in the OR, taking pediatric surgery calls after-hours. It was incredibly demanding work, and long hours, but Dr. Ford, the stern father figure who believed in me, was setting me up to become a competitive candidate for a pediatric surgery fellowship, post-Pitt.

Lab, hospital. Hospital, lab. Early in Year 2, I started getting anxious. After all, I had no categorical position waiting for me where I could finish my last three years of general surgery training. By leaving Brooklyn, I had slammed that door shut.

Again, Dr. Ford advised me just to keep my head down. "If you're doing the work, you'll never have to look for a job," he said. "A job will find you."

"Okay," I said, unconvinced.

In late fall I found myself standing on the buffet line at a national surgical conference next to Dr. Timothy Billiar, the brand-new chair of surgery at Pitt. He asked me how I was doing, how everything was going.

"Good," I said, "except I don't have a job for next year."

Soon as it was out of my mouth, I could just imagine Dr. Ford shaking his head, telling me that that wasn't what he meant by "keeping my head down."

But it turned out to be the right thing—at least, not the wrong thing. At a scheduled meeting after we returned to Pittsburgh, Dr. Billiar told me he had noticed my work ethic and the research I had helped produce in Dr. Ford's lab. He offered me a categorical surgical spot—the chance to stay at Pitt to finish my general surgery training with them! At the time I didn't appreciate how much that would piss off certain people in the surgery department who didn't believe I deserved to be there in the first place. Dr. Billiar was someone who saw something in me that others did not, and I will always be grateful for that.

I said yes to the offer, of course. Best buffet ever.

• • •

If Dr. Henri Ford was the stern father figure, Dr. Edward Barksdale was the kinder, gentler, nurturing supporter. He looked out for me. He provided me with perspective. He made me laugh. When I needed a safe harbor, or made a wrong decision, he was there. He helped me mourn the loss of my grandfather. To get to where I was going, I needed the help of both doctors.

I wrote earlier that I was rough around the edges. Yes, there were sharks in the water, and sometimes they were coming specifically for me, but I also made mistakes. I was quick to boil. I could cry, though privately, a display of vulnerability surgeons are taught to avoid at all costs. I could show frustration. Was I sometimes a little too sure of myself? Dr. Barksdale liked to quote to me his grandmother's saying: "Nothing superior has ever been accomplished except by those who believed they were superior to their circumstance." I told myself I was called to a purpose, not a place, and this happened to be the place to fulfill that purpose. That helped me to develop a sense of personal power. Dr. Barksdale didn't try to change me. "As a result of the chaos, you become better," he offered. "Like Hemingway wrote, 'The world breaks everyone and afterward many are stronger at the broken places.'" I didn't fully understand what he meant, not then.

He told me when I made the wrong clinical decision—such as starting a post-op patient on a diet too early, ordering too many tests, or not getting to the sickest patient first. And though I had done good research, my test-taking ability—going back to those in-service exams in my Brooklyn days—remained awful. He said my technical skills, which I had thought were honed from my experience at Kings County, left something to be desired. That's true of virtually all young surgeons, regardless of race or gender or hand size. But he was frank with me about the racism in medicine, not just for patients but for practitioners, too. "Ala, as a Black doctor, as a Black woman doctor, you have to work harder and be better because you're going to be seen as half as good. And you don't have the pedigree. You have to overcome the lack of one." In other words, I had to overcome my upbringing. In some ways, I was being asked to reach the top of a ladder with missing rungs. I didn't have the foundation others had; nothing would change that and no one cared. I would have to make it without or not make it at all.

At Pitt, I also had to overcome snobbery about my having gone to medical school at Penn State and having been a surgical trainee at Kings County. But the idea that I had to "explain" myself, that I had to prove myself above and beyond anyone there, annoyed the hell out of me. The way I saw it—and still do—many of my colleagues were the ones who needed to adjust, not me. There's a Black woman surgical trainee in your midst: Get over it. The one other Black woman doctor there, Dr. Velma P. Scantlebury*, was a transplant surgeon. She was older, and many of my white surgical colleagues assumed that I was there, in this prestigious, almost-impossible-to-get-into program, because she was my mother. That was the only possible explanation they could wrap their small minds around. It was a shockingly common assumption; people talk, and when word spreads, people assume it's true.

After a while, I just started answering, "Yep, that's my mom."

The fact that I was offered the position to move from the lab to continue my general surgery training at Pitt after showing that I was good in the OR on calls after-hours? That wasn't enough to muffle those who believed I never belonged there in the first place. That it was the head of the department who had personally made the offer? Nope. To the haters, that just made it look suspicious. In fact, it gave them all the more reason to go after me. *Who the hell is this person to take up such a valued spot?* Someone looked at my file and saw my horrendous in-service exam score from Kings County. *What in holy hell did we sign up for?* Word got out. (Word always gets out, right?)

That's how those people score—a friend passed along that snarky

---

*America's first Black woman transplant surgeon.

comment to me—which you could interpret as a dig at all surgeons who trained at Kings County. Or maybe something darker.

Dr. Ford got wind of my awful score. Maybe it was a good thing he hadn't known until then that it was *that* low.

"Okay, you're going to ace the next in-service surgical exam," he said. "Your research and clinical work are stopping. You're studying for the test. That's all you're doing." If I didn't do better on it, Dr. Ford would have a virtually impossible task making the case for me as a superior candidate for a pediatric surgery fellowship, once general surgery training was completed. "We need a great score from you."

"Okay," I said. "Got it."

"Because if you don't, then it doesn't matter how many times you present research at national meetings, or how many papers you write. Without a better score, you'll never get to be a general surgeon, let alone a pediatric surgeon. I'd be doing you a disservice letting you think everything's going to work out."

I was going to need help becoming a better test-taker, so he shipped me off to Buffalo, New York, where his friend, colleague, and mentor, Dr. Eddie Hoover, a Black thoracic surgeon and professor of surgery at SUNY Buffalo Medical School, was going to work with me, along with his residents. Teach me how to study better. How to test better. Test boot camp.

When I arrived in Buffalo, Dr. Hoover's residents stared at me. I assumed they had been prepped on how bad my previous score had been. They must have thought, *Who the hell is she?*

"I told Ala how great you all were," Dr. Hoover told his young doctors, "and that you can teach. She's here from Pitt, and I need you to teach her how to take tests better. Because she's going to be a great pediatric surgeon."

I tried not to get choked up.

They were magic. They taught me to strategize my studying—to "triage," like a doctor does, by focusing first on mastering priority topics before moving on to "lesser" ones. It was all about organization.

Previously, I'd had to figure out things like this on my own. (I got some nuggets of wisdom from my Stanley Kaplan course for the MCATs.) Now, to avoid getting lost, I learned to look at the questions first, before diving into a long reading passage. (Sometimes you didn't even have to read the whole passage!) I learned not to get bogged down on any one question, and to save those tough ones for my deductive reasoning and guessing at the end. I learned how to save time by reading all the answers to a multiple-choice question and ruling out however many I could. If two of the five answers are complete opposites, eliminate the one that is clearly way off. One surgical resident told me that, in a real pinch, statistically the answer is (c) more than any other letter, though I didn't want to rely on that trick. The residents shared study guides they had created, the kind of support that had usually been unavailable to me and many students of color.

I spent two weeks in Buffalo. I stayed at Dr. Hoover's home—me, him, his wife, and their dog. They lived on a farm. In the morning, Dr. Hoover would pull collard greens from his garden, put them in big black plastic garbage bags, and gift them to the nurses in the operating room.

I returned to Pittsburgh with my outline, my study materials, my new confidence. The whole next month leading up to the exam I was in the library all day, every day.

I got 90th percentile.

My score was higher than all but 10 percent of the test-takers that year. Now, when Dr. Ford or anyone else had to advocate for me, the proof was there. This girl from Philly, raised in a single-parent home on public assistance, with no one at her high school believing she could go into medicine, this girl who'd made it to Penn State for undergrad and med school, to Brooklyn to be a warm body to cut and sew, then to Pitt to be a grunt in a lab. This girl sat for the test that was designed to show how aspiring surgeons stacked up against their peers nationally, a measure about as objective as you could get, and she got 90th percentile. In Dr. Ford's words, I had "knocked it out the park."

I finally thought I had control of everything I could control, that no one would mess with me again for reasons having to do with my being Black, or a woman, or, especially, a Black woman.

How naïve.

Another year—now as a general surgeon trainee. I was no longer in the lab. I put my head down; I did the work. I came in the earliest, stayed the latest. I got all my notes done. I made sure there was nothing objective I could be criticized for. The subjective things I couldn't help. Some people just didn't like me. There was nothing I could do about that. But when it came to the things I could control, I made sure no one could find me lacking.

In my journal around that time, I wrote:

Life changing decisions I need to make:

Better environment
Attendings who aren't all out to watch me fail
Residents who have my back
Not be the only one who looks like me
People who appreciate what I bring to the program
Given a fair chance

Support
There's no significant other, but I do have a family
I'm all alone—it's tough sometimes more than others, but still
     tough
This is a hard life and I need some help to sort it out and finish my
     residency

In the months before the end of Year 4, my penultimate year at Pitt and my second as a surgeon there, I applied for a pediatric surgery fellowship for the following year. It was the very reason I'd come to Pitt: They had a good track record of placing their people.

To do pediatric surgery, you first have to complete general surgery, which I was on track to do. Then you apply and hopefully match with a program. If for some reason you don't—which happens about half the time—then you're not considered the cream of the crop, and your chances of *ever* being a pediatric surgeon just dropped significantly. Put it this way: Everyone knows who's been in the match process more than once. Yes, those who are really, truly, obsessively committed will do an extra year or two of another fellowship, maybe in critical care or trauma. Maybe they'll do a year or two of research. That should make them an even *better* doctor, right? But it also adds a year or two or five to your already long career path before you become a pediatric surgeon. Some pediatric surgeons don't become board-certified until they're forty-five years old.

At every institution, there are meetings among senior faculty and administration about who in the program ought to advance. Dr. Ford assured me that he would speak for me. And now, with my superior test score, he had all the ammunition he needed.

To apply for the pediatric surgery fellowship, I also needed recommendations, the most important of which would come from my supervisor, the attending pediatric surgeon. But other surgeons, in different areas, who oversaw me when I did rotations with them, might also weigh in. An attending trauma surgeon asked me to his office. He told me that I had done good work. That I was growing as a doctor. That he could see me growing into the role of chief resident.

One of the best reasons to have faith in yourself is that you never know when you'll need it. And when you do, there it is.

Because what happened next was the first in a series of events of people in power undermining me or trying to undermine me, and me doing all I could to not let that happen.

What that trauma doc subsequently wrote in my report, the one that would be read by the administrators of the pediatric surgery programs to which I was applying, was entirely different from what he told me that day. But I didn't know that yet. I didn't realize that the man was a coward who wouldn't say to my face what he was planning to write.

I found that out when I received a mustard-colored interoffice envelope containing a letter that laid out what happened during my in-person evaluation with him. I was supposed to sign it to indicate that I agreed with the account, then pass it along to the Graduate Medical Education office, where it would go in my file.

But there was a problem. The letter said that I required remediation. That I needed more seasoning. That I might need to repeat the year I was just finishing. That usually only happens if you were negligent—responsible for a patient's death or something equally egregious. If I signed the letter before me, I might be signing away my whole chance at ever matching. Plus, I'd be signing something that was untrue.

I called the offending trauma surgeon. I cussed him out. I called him a liar. He sounded shocked that I was confronting him. He told me to calm down, but I talked right over him. The more he tried to speak, the angrier I became. Finally I said, "I'm hanging up," and I did. Dial tone.

So many of the people in power were not looking out for me. Dr. Ford was, Dr. Barksdale was. Some of the surgeons were, too, but some weren't. I was not their own. I was nothing like their own. Some of these men and women were threatened, whether they admitted it or not, even to themselves. They had to find some way to draw a line to maintain what had always been protected, never challenged.

That night, all I wanted was to sleep and rest my mind. Normally I woke at four to be at the hospital by five. But that morning, when my alarm went off, with Whitney singing the national anthem, I shut it off, turned off my pager, and went back to sleep. I woke again at 6:30 and thought, *I'd be in rounds by now.* I rolled over and fell back asleep. I woke again, at eleven, and called the hospital. "I'm not coming to work," I announced, a pretty self-evident statement since it was practically lunchtime. I offered the person on the other end no explanation why. I knew what a challenge it was for everyone else when a resident didn't show up. But my mental well-being was more important than my presence there.

"When are you coming back?" asked the poor lady on the other end.

"I don't know. Maybe tomorrow." I hung up.

The next day I showed up, on time, as if nothing had happened.

"That's just not what you do," the attending surgeon reprimanded me. I wanted to tell him where he could go, but I refrained. I kept my head down. I was coming close to sabotaging my standing, if not my whole career. On the other hand, I'd already been screwed over for nothing related to my performance.

I called my mentor. Again, like clockwork, Dr. Ford instructed, "Just do the work, Ala. You take care of your patients and let me deal with the rest."

"Why would he do this?" I asked, though I may have screamed it. Cracks in my composure were showing. "Why would he write that in his evaluation? If I have to repeat a surgical residency year, I'll never get a fellowship. That is *not* what he told me to my face!"

"Ala, Ala, calm down—"

"I will *not* calm down! Don't you understand how hard I'm working? I'm so sick of this shit!"

To not match, and to have the reason be that one of my superiors thought I needed a year of remediation, could effectively kill my dream. It just wouldn't fly in a specialty as competitive as pediatric surgery. Later that day, I visited our surgical coordinator, a nonclinician, and told her I would not sign the letter from the trauma surgeon.

"Okay," she said calmly and kindly. "I'll put it in your folder and you don't have to sign it."

Among my young colleagues at Pitt, I was the only one pursuing pediatric surgery that year. The trauma guy had simply decided that *I* was not going to be their recommended candidate. And frankly, it was irrelevant what he thought. He wasn't a pediatric surgeon. Nonetheless, he took it upon himself to make sure that pediatric surgery programs out there knew that, in his opinion, I wouldn't make a good chief surgery resident. Fortunately, pediatric surgery departments want to hear from pediatric surgeons!

I don't know what exactly was said to whom, but I was never again approached to sign that paper. It was never submitted. Maybe the trauma surgeon recanted. The idea that I would have a critique of my ability lurking somewhere, just waiting to undermine me, was moot (though you can tell I'm still mad about it to this day). I won the battle, but going to work at an institution where so many people quietly resented me was often miserable.

I *could* have been brought up on charges of insubordination—yelling at various superiors in frustration, taking a day off of work without cause—but I never was. Maybe those in charge realized I had every reason to be furious.

The two individuals who most saw me through and helped me thrive at Pitt took care of me like their own. They shared a bond not just with me but with each other.

Henri and Edward became best friends at age seventeen. They met in New York City at an enrichment program for underprivileged kids. Henri was born and raised in Haiti, Ed in Lynchburg, Virginia. Neither of Ed's parents went to college; his mother didn't graduate from high school. Henri was the more outgoing and charismatic of the two, Ed the more philosophical. But they were both headstrong teenaged boys, maybe even a bit arrogant, "with that testosterone bravado." They wanted to change the world. They felt they could.

Henri went to Princeton. Ed went to Yale.

They fell mostly out of touch over the next four years but reconnected at Harvard Medical School. They still wanted to change the world, "to build skill sets that would allow us to empower and help grow others, and ourselves." After medical school, they again went their separate ways, this time for a decade, until they came back together again at the University of Pittsburgh Medical Center. Henri arrived first and convinced Ed that they could "build that world. Let's make a difference."

When I arrived at Pitt, these two men saw me as someone raw and green, lacking intellectual sophistication. But they also saw me as an individual who could develop into something special; maybe they even saw something of themselves in me. Others—and I don't mean that as a euphemism for white people—may have just seen in me what was unsophisticated and lacking. Henri and Ed saw the rough spots, but they knew that a few chisels were all it would take to get at the essence beneath. The more they chiseled, the more I could move.

Dr. Ford—Henri—completed general surgery to train at Children's Hospital of Pittsburgh. Dr. Barksdale—Ed—completed his training at Massachusetts General Hospital and then left to train in pediatrics at Children's Hospital Medical Center in Cincinnati. He was the first African American pediatric surgery fellow there, and for his first three months the nurses never acknowledged him. They thought he had to be a medical student. They didn't take his orders. Think about the indifference and belittling, for someone who was board-certified and had been an attending surgeon at famed Mass General. Not that his is a remotely unusual story among Black physicians, especially Black male physicians, all of whom have their own depressingly similar tales. Studying late, forgot your ID in your car, Security doesn't believe you're a resident at the hospital, cops get called and arrest you. Maybe handcuffs because you got "belligerent." That sort of thing. Not in the 1950s but the 1990s. The 2000s. The 2010s. Today.

Ed was one of the first Black men to be trained as a pediatric surgeon in the U.S. Same with Henri.

I keep saying I had rough edges because I did. Maybe I was needy. Maybe I needed love. Maybe I was a girl in a woman's body, which is not the best dynamic in a male-dominated world like surgery. I had to learn to fit in, and not everyone wanted me to. Maybe I lacked maturity in certain ways. When things got rough at Pitt, I would call Dr. B. to talk me down. I trusted him. I trusted them both. But I was careful not to be a burden. They had their own challenges establishing themselves in academic surgery.

When I checked myself into Health Services in medical school after the episode with the child molester in the amphitheater, I was surrounded by so many people who were broken, and I wanted to get out of there as quickly as possible. I observed them as if they were so unlike me. But they *were* me. I was broken in places. Now I had to fill those places with gold epoxy. So that people saw gold, not the cracks. I had flaws, ones that would not disappear; I had to recognize those flaws, adapt because of them. I needed to be as honest and self-aware as possible to get where I wanted to go.

Henri and Ed were hell-bent on getting me to match—but also in preparing me for all the things I would have to combat in becoming a surgeon. We didn't have the network others in the medical establishment enjoyed—in getting into medical school, thriving there, matching at the best hospitals—but we did what we could. Henri had enlisted his mentor, Dr. Eddie Hoover, to help me to become a better test-taker. And beyond any informal network of established Black doctors helping younger Black doctors, there was a formal one, too. The Society of Black Academic Surgeons, established in 1989, was (and remains) a mentoring organization and a valuable resource. At meetings, it was thrilling to see all these residents and medical students who looked like me. We talked about what it was like on the wards, about our attendings, about upcoming exams. We shared intel on those hospitals that were, or subtly were *not*, welcoming to residents of color. There were panel discussions where the senior surgeons outlined the skills we would need to survive. *Be nonconfrontational. Arrive early, stay late. Give 150 percent. Don't complain; the generation before you had it way harder.* Some of the younger doctors were bold enough to get up to the microphone and ask questions, and the senior doctors were only too eager to share how tough it had been for them. It was a place for collaborative projects and discussing one's work. I presented the results of multiple research papers there.

Yep: Now I, Ala Stanford, finally had a support system! My medical village. I had people specifically looking out for me, though not always publicly. The playing field of life that so many Black Americans are born into is not level; often you didn't know all the rules of the game, so whether or not you could play it was already tilted away from you. Now, finally, I had some people in my corner who could teach me the rules. They were going to do what they could, *within the system*, to help me.

Dr. Henri Ford became a world-renowned pediatric surgeon. He will always be larger than life to me. Dr. Edward Barksdale became a world-renowned pediatric surgeon, as well, and he, too, will always be larger than life. They didn't have to take a chance on me, but they did, and now I had to pay it forward.

Matthew, a pediatric dental resident at Pitt, and I met during my fourth year there. We lived in the same apartment building, a beautiful old schoolhouse that had been converted into loft apartments. Our courtship was a bit of a blur—both of us so busy with the demands of our programs—but Nick, the building handyman, filled each of us in on the goings-on of the other. Matt was a cyclist, and we watched the Tour de France together, and I noted that my favorite part was when the peloton rode past endless fields of sunflowers. Soon after, I returned from work to find, sitting atop my coffee table, a cyclist's plastic water bottle with a sunflower in it. Who had been in my apartment? It was from Matt, with matchmaker Nick letting him in. Normally I would have been livid. But it showed that someone was thinking about me, so I couldn't be upset. I felt special and seen. Matt proposed early—and unexpectedly—at the start of my fifth and final year, at the Carnegie Museum of Art. I said yes.

As difficult as it is to match by yourself, it's that much more difficult if you're a couple, both hoping to be at the same institution or at least the same geographical area. Hospitals will often accommodate; if they really want one of the two, they'll try to find a place in the other person's discipline, too.

I applied to all the major programs in pediatric surgery, including Boston Children's, Cincinnati Children's, Children's Hospital of Philadelphia (CHOP), and St. Christopher's Hospital for Children ("St. Chris," also in Philly). Pitt had a great pediatric program but (a) the previous year they had picked an internal candidate and were unlikely to do that two years running, and (b) I'd exhausted my time there.

I got an interview at St. Chris, but then I found out that my former superior at Kings County, the chain-smoker who had put his hands on me, had recently taken a position there as a staff pediatric surgeon.

When I told a colleague about it, she said, "Don't interview there. You're better than that." To top it off, when St. Chris sent the letter for my interview date, on the bottom of the letter were four handwritten words: "Don't interview. She's dumb." With his initials. I was unsure if it was sent by accident or on purpose.

I declined what should have been an incredible opportunity.

Fortunately, there were other places that wanted to speak with me. On the interview trail, I ran into other candidates. While in Toronto to interview at the Hospital for Sick Children, another top-tier pediatric institution, I met a Harvard-trained resident from Mass General. We chatted about our backgrounds and recent experience, and at one point she said something about "our chief clinic."

"What's that?" I asked.

"It's for the uninsured. They're able to come into a clinic and get care. It's supervised by the chief residents."

"But chief residents aren't board-certified yet," I pointed out. "What goes on at the clinic?"

"We take care of patients. We operate. We run the whole thing."

"But if you're not board-certified, who—what—gives you the authority to take care of these folks?" *Is it because they're poor?* I wanted to add.

"It's the Harvard way," she said. "And if not for us, they wouldn't have a place to go."

"Let me get this straight," I said, trying not to betray anger. I laid it out slowly so that I didn't get any details wrong. "Residents who are not completely or optimally trained . . . not board-certified . . . take care of poor people who don't have insurance . . . and then Harvard justifies it by saying, 'Well, at least we're taking care of the poor.'"

Yeah, she didn't take kindly to the way I put it. At Kings County, we took care of everyone, regardless of their ability to pay. We didn't separate out the insured from the uninsured. And our top doctors were all board-certified. The way she described her clinic, it was basically trainees practicing on patients unsupervised. This is how it was back then. Hopefully now it has changed, with more oversight. Uninsured and underinsured also deserve more attention to detail with their care delivery.

The woman and I argued. They were able to do it that way, she explained, because the residents were under the supervision of an attending surgeon who was always "within arm's length." There to provide guidance, when needed. So it wasn't, you know, *illegal*. But I found it not just dubious but patronizing. Like: *These people are getting something even though we're treating them as if they're not worthy of optimal care.*

"Ala, I don't know why you're being like this," said the resident, not the first person to feel my wrath. "And if it's a very interesting case that no one's seen before, then it gets moved to the wing with the private payer patients, because now it's a teaching case. So then they get the expertise of the attendings!"

This is how it was back then. My eyes were opening up more, bit by bit.

Right around the time I was set to graduate from Pitt in 2004, I received terrible news from Chicago: Heather, my best friend from childhood, the one I told almost everything to, had been diagnosed with lymphoma. It had started with a sore throat, then the sore throat wouldn't go away, and after a few tests they came up with the awful diagnosis. All I could do from another city was be there by phone when Heather needed me, and visit Chicago when I could.

The bitter and the sweet: Shortly thereafter, in June, I became the first Black woman to complete her general surgery training at Pitt.

Years later, I forged a friendship with the Black woman resident a couple years behind me at Pitt, who had often acted cold toward me. "When I was at Pitt you decided we were not going to be friends," I pointed out. "You decided to side with everyone else."

"I should have been there for you," she admitted. "Rather than speak up, I was with the group. People treated you like shit." She apologized. "I don't know how you made it through that."

For whatever reason, and despite my resentment, I was ready to accept her apology.

Actually, that's not true. I know *exactly* why I accepted her apology: because I understood her. She had just been trying to protect herself. She was a Black woman trying to make it as a surgeon. You do whatever you have to.

8

THANK YOU FOR YOUR SERVICE

I matched—I matched!

And not just any place: Little Ala got into Cincinnati Children's, one of the top pediatric surgery programs in the country. A beautiful moment. I ran down the hall of the pediatric surgery suite in Pittsburgh to Ben, surgical fellow and trusted friend. We hugged, I cried, we screamed together. Dr. Barksdale had trained at Cincinnati (though he felt he hadn't always been treated well there). And Cincinnati did something that not all pediatric programs did: transplantation, for kidney, liver, and intestinal bowel. Dr. Alberto Peña had just come there from New York to build the colorectal program; he had more or less invented the procedure to correct anorectal malformations. It happens in roughly one in 2,500 kids—something one is born with and often needs to be fixed within twenty-four to forty-eight hours after delivery. Depending on how intricate the anomaly, some children can wait until they're six months. Kids came in from all over the country and the world for treatment.

All of my attendings at Cincinnati were great teachers, but Dr.

Peña showed me a certain level of concern, and I wondered if it was because we were both underrepresented. He was Mexican. He had an accent. He told me, "You will be my eyes" and "I will teach you everything you need to know."

He did teach me a lot, but I wasn't really his eyes so much as his hands. When he arrived in Cincinnati, his Ohio medical license application was pending, which was required to operate—never mind that he was licensed in New York, or that he was a master surgeon, or that he had trained thousands of young doctors. I would scrub and he would stand directly behind me and tell me what to do when it came to the complicated parts. Imagine how brilliant a surgeon you have to be to operate without touching the patient. And he kept to his word, teaching me how to operate with elegance, how every move should be intentional, orchestrated. It wasn't a surprise that he loved classical music.

The state license eventually came, and Dr. Peña's legend only grew. People flew him all over the world to operate on children and sometimes adults with the most complex anatomy. The basement of his Cincinnati home was crammed with gifts from grateful families. In one of the many foreign countries where he operated, the hospital administration arranged for a string quartet to play for the duration of the operation.

"The eyes see only what the mind suspects," Dr. Peña liked to say. That is, you won't know to look out for aberrant anatomy, for example, if you haven't first read about it in a textbook or done the procedure previously.

Among the many things I learned at Cincinnati was transplantation. I did it occasionally, not often. It's a grueling odyssey that makes a long surgery even longer. With kids, you're especially likely to travel personally to procure the organ. Someone unfortunately has died, and kids are on a waiting list for organs that match. Sometimes I would do the procurement with another surgeon, which meant we would get on a Learjet or a helicopter to wherever the child whose organs were being harvested was being kept alive. You bring a permit stating that you can procure the organ. You land, race to the hospital, and there's someone taking the child's heart, someone else taking the liver, someone taking the intestine. Whoever is in line for the kidney might be taking one or both. The on-staff anesthesiologist is keeping the patient alive while you remove the organ. You don't worry about how much the donor is bleeding because they're going to die, but you need still to be respectful of their body. It's emotionally harrowing, if you let it be.

Then it's a race against time. You flush the organ with the right solutions to keep it viable. You put it on ice in a cooler. You take the private jet or helicopter back home, then race from the airport to the hospital to the OR, where the recipient patient is open and waiting.

Transplant surgery is exacting and exhausting. When you're removing the organ, you'd better not cut a vein too short or you'll find it impossible to sew it into the recipient. And I didn't particularly enjoy when the flight home was turbulent (it always seemed as if we were flying in bad weather). On the other hand, it also got me out of call at the hospital—a break from the litany of appendectomies and circumcisions and abscess drainings.

As happens in all medicine, and especially in subspecialties like oncology and pediatric surgery, there is a lot to endure emotionally. Every time you operate on a child with malrotation and midgut volvulus, to take an example, time is critical. You hold your breath until you open them. You exhale when you see viable intestines, or you shriek silently when you see the bowel is dead and you have to tell the family that this otherwise perfect baby for whom they were waiting and dreaming for nine months is about to die.

I tried to save a two-year-old who ended up in the trauma bay for blunt force trauma. The family watched us try to resuscitate him. The boy died. I can still hear the father screaming and punching walls, the mother wailing.

A high school junior born with an imperforate anus came in; her classmates teased her, saying she looked pregnant, and worse, called her "Stinky" because she leaked stool during the day. The operation I performed changed her life, and it was gratifying to see her parents so involved in her success. The young woman and I would maintain a relationship through her college years. She called me when she had her first baby.

The last year of this whole, long, grueling, nine-year process—*nine years!*—of post–medical school surgical training was capped off by job-hunting. Early in 2006, while still at Cincinnati, I was excited for an upcoming interview at DuPont Hospital for Children in Delaware. Then a friend and supporter, one of the attending Cincinnati surgeons, landed another interview for me, at CHOP, Children's Hospital of Philadelphia. One morning, not long after securing that interview, I was outside the OR, ready to perform surgery. I found myself standing beside another of the attending surgeons and I mentioned my Philadelphia interview.

Three days later, right before heading to Philly, I got a voice message. CHOP couldn't see me. I called to find out what had happened. The response was disturbingly vague. The position they thought they had was no longer available.

That's it?

When I reported the disappointing news to the supportive surgeon who had enthusiastically set up the interview, he too was confused. And annoyed. He asked me to describe what happened. There wasn't much to report. "They just said they didn't want to see me anymore," I said.

He shook his head, disbelieving. "It makes no sense. They were excited about you coming. I *know* it." He paused. "Did you tell anyone about the interview?"

I thought for a moment. Oh, yeah. I had mentioned it to his colleague.

My friend shook his head. "I'm sure he said something to them."

But why would our staff surgeon want to undermine my post-fellowship employment?

Wait, I thought. *What else had I told him that he might use to sabotage me?* If this was happening again, then it must be me, right? Was I an impostor? I was devastated. Embarrassed. I couldn't help but wonder about what the CHOP leadership had been told and what they were now spreading throughout their hospital about me. CHOP was (and is) arguably the best children's hospital in the world. They had offered me an interview for the fellowship spot, so they knew who I was.

But damn. Just like that, the possibility was gone.

I still had the DuPont interview, but DuPont was not CHOP. I had to wonder how—not if, *how*—this would be taken from me, too. I put on a fake smile and headed to Delaware . . . and the interview went very well! They liked me, I liked them—and they made me an offer! I just needed to get my Delaware medical license and we'd be good.

Ala Stanford, all set to graduate, finishing up a highly regarded pediatric surgery fellowship at Cincinnati Children's Hospital, gets offered a position at DuPont Hospital for Children, in Wilmington, Delaware. Something to look forward to. How exciting!

Matthew submitted his resignation from his group practice in Cincinnati; DuPont was looking into pediatric dental opportunities for him in their system. We put all our savings, fifteen thousand dollars, toward the purchase of a house in Wilmington, not far from the hospital. The house had a big, bright bay window in the kitchen. There was a yard, a double garage, relatively new appliances. Four bedrooms. On the walls below and above the banister leading from the first to the second floor, the owners had hung drawings that their kids had done at different ages. I could imagine our own future there, with a big family. The date for the house closing was set.

Then a call came from the chief of surgery at DuPont. "We don't think we can use you," he said.

What?

I had the offer letter in hand. I had accepted the job.

"I'm sorry," he said. They were officially rescinding.

When I hung up, I couldn't breathe. Every dollar Matthew and I had saved had gone into the deposit on the house, perfectly situated near the hospital with a pediatric surgical opening that I was supposed to fill. My husband had quit his dental practice. I was graduating in three months, after investing nine years of my life *on top of medical school on top of college* in achieving my dream.

Now I had no job. I figured I'd try to find another position in the state, or at least close to the new house. I'd still need to get credentialed to practice in Delaware.

The interview was in-person. I flew from Cincinnati and made my way to the Delaware State Medical Board headquarters. Across the desk was my interviewer, a licensing doctor who served in the military, a Black man who informed me that he was shipping off to Iraq the very next day. We talked for a bit. "Dr. Stanford, I think you'll be a great addition to the state of Delaware," he said, "but one thing in your file really stands out, and I wanted to ask you about it."

"What is it?"

"What happened when you went before the disciplinary board?"

I must have misheard. "I'm sorry?"

"The disciplinary board?"

"What are you talking about?"

He pulled a sheet from my file.

"There's a letter, an addendum actually, no more than a paragraph, from one of your attending surgeons in Cincinnati. It says a formal committee was called. That as a pediatric surgery fellow you were put on academic probation. And that you need remedial teaching. And that if it were up to him, he wouldn't let you graduate."

WHAT?

Once again, I had trouble breathing.

"But the three letters of recommendation in your file," the interviewer continued, "not one of them mentions anything about probation or anything close to what this other person says. They're all glowing. So I'm trying to figure out what's true."

My head was spinning. My heart was pounding. I managed to push a few words out. "I've never been on probation. No such hearing ever happened. That is . . . completely untrue."

Why would a person in my program say that? What would make him lie like that? A *provable* lie?

The interviewer removed the offending letter—addendum—from my file and held it out to me. I took the paper and stared at the words, dumbfounded—or whatever word means dumbfounded times a thousand.

Observing my reaction, the doctor sat back with a glum look and shook his head. "I see this crap all the time," he said, "particularly with Black folks. I've seen other young Black physicians torpedoed by a combination of doubt and suspicion from white superiors. It ruins people's careers before they even get started—and they never know what happened."

Some senior doctor or other authority figure puts something undermining in the application. Sometimes it's subtle. Sometimes it's not subtle at all. And the qualified applicant never figures out why they keep getting turned down, or having scheduled interviews mysteriously canceled. Some of them finally give up.

"Take this paper," the interviewer said, holding out the letter, "and when you get to your home institution, go to your Graduate Medical Education office. Show this to them. I'm going to recommend that you get your license for the state, and I wish you the best."

Out in the parking lot, I cried. And cried. I didn't know which feeling was stronger—confusion? Rage? Disgust? I couldn't believe I had worked so closely with this person in authority who was out to derail my career and life. How many times did I have to go through this shit? Powerful gatekeepers flat-out lying about me, hard-won opportunities dashed? How many people out there were aiming to keep me down?

I could have so easily succumbed to cynicism and misanthropy.

These experiences, one after the other, seemed designed to teach me that no matter how much people smiled at me, hugged me, or encouraged me to confide in them . . . no matter how supportive they may have acted, the moment it suited them they'd stab me in the back.

Yet I would not lose faith. In fact, I had actually been lucky. Had my interviewer not been a sympathetic Black man; had he not been kind enough to give me the actual letter; had I arrived a day later, after he had shipped off for Iraq, and someone else had reviewed my file, someone who didn't share with me what had been falsely and maliciously inserted into my file . . . my career might never have unfolded the way it ultimately did.

The question that confused me most: Why did the surgeon express, *in writing*, that I was on academic probation? That was a verifiable claim, not an opinion. If someone thinks you need remedial teaching—which can happen—it's an opinion. But to say that I was on probation? That's either true or it's not, and it wasn't. Now I held concrete proof that the attending surgeon had lied.

Back in Cincinnati I showed the Graduate Medical Education officer what I had discovered. It had cost me a job offer, and probably the interview in Philadelphia, too. Maybe it was grounds for a lawsuit.

To his credit, the GME officer was horrified. "Well, Ala, what do you want us to do?"

Why was he asking me? I wanted *him* to outline the steps they would take to correct this awful, demeaning situation—

Then the realization came. I started to see the light. Maybe this is why people in power get away with this "crap," as the military doctor had put it.

The man who was sabotaging my career was also the man who would sign—or not sign—the certificate that verified that I had graduated. Without that, I would have trouble getting a job as a surgeon anywhere. I needed to pass my general surgery boards, oral and written. Mind you, young surgeons have failed those exams and still been allowed to move forward—but for me, in my circumstances, with my skin color and gender: *If you fail those tests, Ala,* I told myself, *you're done.*

But once I passed my general surgery boards (I could study for my pediatric surgery boards later), there would be nothing else to talk about or hold me back. I would be board-certified. Everyone knew I worked hard, every day. That I took care of my patients. That I was good in the OR. I had killed no patients. I never felt as if I wasn't good enough, but this creep was challenging that self-belief. Once I passed my boards, there would be no legitimate reason to keep me from graduating and holding me back from being a surgeon, somewhere. He would have a really hard time in my last two months in the program coming up with a case for why I couldn't graduate. And if this asshole *did* try to hold me back after I passed my boards, well, now I had proof that he had a history of dishonestly trying to stop me from succeeding. Likely I wasn't the only one he'd done this to.

"Leave it alone," I said to the GME officer, finally—wiser, sadder, madder. "I'm about to graduate. I just want to get out of here. I want to figure out what's next. This is a horrible situation, and I don't deserve this—but no. Don't say anything to him."

I absolutely wanted to curse out the surgeon who had done me wrong. But I didn't. I had learned from the similar incident at Pitt with the trauma surgeon that I needed to be strategic, not reactive and emotional.

When the chair of surgery learned of the "incident" (people talk), he was horrified. He came to me, but I had little patience for anyone's sympathy.

"God, can I just make it to the end of the school year?" I told him.

I took the general surgery boards, written and oral. I passed. I had fulfilled the requirements. There were no red flags.

As we approached graduation, I shared with some of my colleagues that I had no job waiting. (Might as well admit it to them—they would learn sooner or later. Again: People talk.) My chief of surgery offered me a job to stay at Cincinnati and work with one of my favorite surgeons. But it was for about half of what pediatric surgeons earn coming out of there. There was no pay line for the position, and the surgery chief was kindly creating what he could with nondiscretionary funds. I appreciated the effort and the offer, but I didn't want to stay at a place where a high-ranking colleague had totally screwed me over. It was Pitt all over again.

Instead of being one of the happiest days of my life, graduation was bittersweet. Jubilation was replaced by sadness. No job, no home, embarrassed, out of money. Matthew also unemployed.

My peers all knew that I had suffered some injustice but not the details. They knew that Matthew and I had plunked our life savings on a house in another city where no job awaited. Many of my colleagues wrote me supportive letters and cards. *This is not who we are. I'm so sorry you had to go through this.*

There was one redeeming moment. At the graduation ceremony, someone—an attending surgeon, a parent, a spouse—would get to make a remark about each graduate. In commenting about me, Dr. Victor Garcia, one of my attendings, said "racism and bias are alive and well in surgical training." You could hear a pin drop. Offstage, my mother loudly added, "You don't mess with God's children," and then, for good measure, threw in a verse about the Lord's vengeance.

After graduation, with nowhere to go, I sought a position at D.C. Children's. I inquired at other places. Finally, three months later, I was offered a slot at Temple University Children's Medical Center, a relatively new hospital in my hometown.

All this complication and heartache because an unsolicited letter from a surgeon in my pediatric surgery department was sent to the Delaware medical board and included in my file. What a coward! But I had made one request: that my chair of surgery write the American Board of Surgery, instructing them that this surgeon should never be allowed to write a letter of recommendation on my behalf. I would halt the saboteur before he could act.

Yet, as I wrote earlier, I felt lucky. I was grateful for my parents and grandparents and brother and husband, my extended family and mentors and friends, for building me back up when needed. I felt as if God had protected me, particularly on the day of my interview for the state license in Delaware. A Black physician sitting across the table, about to ship off to Iraq, his last day in the office. In a way, my application was his last duty before leaving. He saw the letter in my file. He recognized right away that something was off, given all the other complimentary reports. He gave me the opportunity to address it. I was fortunate. I was glad for God's hand.

But what about those other people? Those who can't understand why they've been denied a license or a job offer? Those staying up at night blaming themselves, wondering where they went wrong? Those who are too naïve and trusting to believe that all it takes is a few racists or misogynists or racist misogynists in powerful positions, or maybe just one, to damn them at any key turn?

9

THE LITTLE ONES

At Temple Children's I operated primarily on newborns and young people up to age twenty-one.

Every patient matters because every patient matters to someone, but the newborns and the premature infants always gave me the most pause. They have no reserve—not much blood, immature immune system, fragile respiratory system—so you have to get it right. There is often no second chance. When a baby is born, we all expect it to be perfect—and then it turns out that something is wrong and just hours into their new surroundings they need help. The parents are expecting to hold the baby and take pictures. Mom wants to feed it. Now, instead, they're in the maternity wing without their baby, or in the NICU waiting room, the last waiting room anyone wants to be in, praying that their baby is going to be all right—to survive. In some ways, as pediatric surgeon, you become the parent for the parents.

Each and every surgery I performed felt to the patient and their family like some of the most stressful hours—often *the* most stressful—they had ever endured, even when it was a routine procedure. For me, though, the OR was a place where I could focus and not think about my own health issues. Because in the fall of 2006, I was having difficulties myself with conceiving. My estrogen levels were normal and an exploratory laparoscopy had concluded that my anatomy was normal, too.

I started medication to stimulate my ovaries at the right time. About a week and a half later, when my levels were optimal, the fertility doctor did an ultrasound, and my eggs were retrieved for in vitro fertilization. When the time was right again, the now fertilized eggs were transferred back, and Matthew and I crossed our fingers.

I visited the fertility doctor regularly to have blood drawn and make sure things were proceeding smoothly. But I soon grew tired of the office, sitting in the clinic waiting room with the same women, all of us wearing the identical am-I-ever-going-to-get-pregnant? expression. Some of them were there alone, some with stressed partners. Fortunately, I could draw my own blood, so at home I tied the tourniquet around my upper arm, used the butterfly needle and vacutainer with Matt, and one of us would drop the sample off at the lab. Those times were stressful as hell; I was also injecting myself with fertility medication multiple times per day. It hurt. I had bruises. Matt wondered if it was all worth it. My emotions were all over the place and, to complicate things, I was surrounded all day at work by babies. Sometimes it was comforting to hear the infant cries. Sometimes it was painful.

After a combined five tries of insemination and IVF, I finally got pregnant, with twins. We were so grateful—until, around Week 8, when I miscarried one of them. It had happened late enough that we had already heard two heartbeats, already had pictures of Twin A and Twin B, already began choosing names. The nurse told me without telling me, and I had trouble digesting the news.

"What do you mean, 'I hear only one heartbeat'?" I snapped, accusingly.

"Please talk to the doctor," said the technician, stepping quickly from the room.

When the doctor entered, she said, "Sometimes, one of the babies doesn't make it."

Immediately after the doctor's visit I returned to work. "Like a Star" by Corinne Bailey Rae was playing on the car radio; even now I can't listen to that song without it taking me back to that day.

It took me a long time to accept the loss. In my journal I wrote to my lost child: "I'm sorry I couldn't protect you. I am supposed to protect you."

I was terrified that I would lose the other twin.

A couple of weeks later, on a fall afternoon on Martha's Vineyard, I experienced spotting and cramps. Terrified, I told Matt, "We gotta get off the island and back to my doctor!" We cut our vacation short and began the trek home. I was sure I had already lost the second baby.

As soon as we landed we headed straight to the ob-gyn office at my hospital, a more affluent facility in the suburbs of Philadelphia. It was Friday, and the office was closing in half an hour, but I had called ahead to tell them I would be there in time. Though I was a patient of the group practice, I was still early enough in my pregnancy that I had not yet met all the doctors. In the waiting room, when I heard the doctor's voice, I looked up and felt hopeful. He was standing at the check-in desk. I could see him. I was sitting right in the waiting area. And then I heard his impatient tone. "I thought we were done for the day," he said, irritated. "Does she have an appointment?"

"Nope," the receptionist responded.

"What are we, a walk-in clinic now? We don't take walk-ins." The volume at which he spoke suggested he didn't care that I could hear him, as both he and the receptionist looked in my direction. I was the only patient in the waiting area. Maybe that was the point.

I was too agitated by his tone, and too scared for my baby, to appreciate just then how much the moment echoed those when Kamau and I, as kids, would go to the ER for help that did not exactly rise to the level of a medical emergency. Then, as now, we were made to feel unwelcome by people who were trained and supposedly driven to help those in need.

That echo is always there.

I left the office in tears and went to the ER, in the same hospital. Everyone there knew me. They attended to me right away. The on-call ob-gyn checked the baby's heartbeat, did a pelvic exam, and reassured me that the spotting and cramps weren't perilous but likely the passing of the contents of my miscarriage. Everything was okay, he reassured me.

People talk. Word got out. *You hear how the on-staff pediatric surgeon got turned away from her doctor in her own hospital?* There were apologies all over—blah blah blah. I didn't care about the apology. I was a pregnant woman in distress and an ob-gyn basically told me to kick rocks. Why? Because it was late on a Friday and he might miss his tennis date? I won't make generalizations about why I, in particular, was treated—or not treated—the way I was. I didn't identify myself as a doctor. I shouldn't have had to. And what if I were white?*

After being at Temple University for a year, I was named director of the Center for Minority Health & Health Disparities at the medical school. I led community outreach and set up education workshops about health conditions prevalent in North Philadelphia (cardiovascular disease, diabetes, maternal health needs including prenatal care, postpartum care, and breastfeeding). While in my third trimester, I was one of several pregnant women celebrating at a community baby shower, held near the former Budd Factory in North Philly, and I couldn't help but notice, with gratitude and also sadness and anger, how different my pregnancy was from those of many of the women in the room. The shower was one of our outreach activities, a great opportunity to discuss prenatal and postnatal care. As the director, I could have had a staff member lead the conversation, but I thought

---

*I now wear my ID badge for every doctor's appointment for myself, and also when I accompany my parents and children to doctor's appointments. It sometimes makes a difference. I shouldn't have to.

it would be more persuasive for me to do so, now that I was a pregnant Black woman. I could sense the women were antsy. They paid
occasional attention to me but they were clearly anxious to get to the
resource tables, where representatives from community organizations,
nonprofits, and Temple University Hospital sported all kinds of free
stuff: powdered formula, car seats, diapers, bottles, strollers, gift cards,
grocery vouchers, and so much more that most of these women did not
have, nor the money to buy it.

Maybe the second thing about the whole pregnancy experience I
was most grateful for was the excellent health insurance I had through
Temple. How many people have that?

Two months later my first child was born, via C-section, after almost two days in labor not progressing. Ellison Matthew, named for
the author of *Invisible Man*. Had we not lost Ellison's twin, she would
have been Ella Grace, because my entire life up to that point had been
powered, more than anything else, by the grace of God.

With my new position at the Center for Minority Health & Health
Disparities, I was asked to speak to the Allegheny West Foundation,
a nonprofit that works to improve housing, education, employment,
health care, and other opportunities for people in need in that part of
Pennsylvania. It went well, and the fact that I was a Philly native made
my message resonate even more. When I received another call to speak,
this time at a local high school, I was thrilled to accept. I was becoming
more and more interested in exploring disparities in opportunities and
outcomes. I thought of how my own life had been transformed when
I saw that well-dressed, upbeat Black woman doctor when I was eight,
and how I wanted to grow up to be like her.

"We're not paying you to be a motivational speaker," my boss told
me when I mentioned the upcoming event. "We're paying you to operate."

Yeah, well, I could do both. I *had* to do both—as a Black woman
doctor, I owed it, particularly to the young people I could reach, to

demonstrate that we were not so different. To show them that we were from the same place. That their minds, like mine, could be their way to more opportunities. That their dreams were within reach. I needed to model what a pediatric surgeon looked and acted like, while also shining light on some of the true causes behind disparities in health care.

In April of 2007 I flew to Chicago for the annual Society of Black Academic Surgeons meeting, to hear my fellow surgeons, including the very impressive Dr. S. Allan Counter, a neurology professor from Harvard, speak about the latest issues. It was a black-tie event and I invited Heather and her husband, Kendrick, to attend as my guests. Heather looked good, not as frail as she had on previous occasions over the last few years. It was wonderful to see her and Kendrick dancing together and happy. The next morning, as they drove me to the airport, Heather sitting with me in the backseat, she faced me, then placed her hands atop her head and shifted her hair back and forth, just enough. It was a wig. "Wanna see?" she asked.

"Absolutely!"

She removed her wig. She once had the most beautiful hair of anyone I'd ever met, and now she had the most beautiful bald head. We laughed.

"Your reaction is so different from Sannah's," said Heather about her firstborn, who was now eight. Heather chuckled. "When I removed the wig for her, she said, 'Don't *ever* take that off again.'"

We burst out laughing like we were teenagers again.

Not long after that, while attending another gathering of doctors, I had a much nastier encounter. At a medical conference in Florida, I ran into one of the surgeons who had tried to destroy my dream, the one from Cincinnati Children's. I made a beeline to him. In the years since, I had heard more about his reputation for screwing over almost every resident of color that came through his program.

"Why did you do that?" I asked, barely containing my fury. I figured he knew what "that" meant. He'd better.

"At the time I thought it was the right thing to do," he said. "If I had to do it again . . . I probably wouldn't have."

What? I couldn't help but hear it as an admission, his way of saying that "at the time" he was protecting the old guard, the system, some bullshit. These guys were so used to walking on water.

A year or so after that, the surgeon was no longer with the institution at Cincinnati. I don't know if he was fired, resigned, or was pushed out but he was no longer there. That didn't stop him from landing another job. It usually doesn't. Someone's trash is another person's treasure and enjoys new benefits though they don't deserve it.

My brilliant, beautiful friend Heather, she of the gorgeous smile and the luscious hair, originally in pigtails, who I giggled with and double-dutched with, died of complications from lymphoma on July 7, 2008. She had undergone a stem cell transplant four months before, and we'd all held out hope that it would work, after years of sickness.

My faith helped me to stay positive—that and Dr. Ford's eternal admonition to "keep your head down and do the work." Especially in trying times I could see how much that advice helped. I kept my head down, and so did Matthew, while we were raising our young son. Temple Children's closed, but I landed on my feet. In the summer and fall of 2008, I accepted two more hospital appointments—as director of Pediatric Surgical Services at Abington Memorial Hospital, just outside of Philly, and as attending pediatric surgeon at St. Christopher's.

In March 2010, after another high-risk pregnancy, I gave birth to two more boys, Robeson and Langston. You could say Robeson was named for the great singer and activist, the namesake of the cultural center where I worked at Penn State, but really it was to honor a family friend, Staff Sergeant Paul Robeson Jackson, a member of an elite Army Special Forces unit who had passed away less than a year earlier during a helicopter training exercise, aged thirty-three. I called his mother to make sure it was all right for us to name our son for hers.

Langston was named for Langston Hughes, the poet who had meant so much to me, whose beautiful words I had inscribed under the mural I painted in college. Ellison, Robeson, and Langston. There were quite a few things, increasingly, that Matthew and I did not agree on, but naming our sons for extraordinary Black men was not one of them.

In his very first days, Langston had neonatal jaundice. The pediatrician, knowing I was a doctor, asked me, "What do you think?"

What do I *think? You're the doctor now!* You *tell* me!

Of course, I knew how fortunate I was. We all were. Neonatal jaundice is easily treatable. For all the failures and inequities in the American health care system, certain conditions and defects—tongue-tie, pyloric stenosis, Hirschsprung's disease, imperforate anus, esophageal atresia, to name just a few—are capably and routinely dealt with soon after birth in this country. There was no question that Langston would be coming home with us.

That kind of service is not true everywhere. Just a few months earlier, a large contingent from my hospital had flown to Haiti to offer medical care and surgical procedures; because of my high-risk pregnancy, I wasn't able to join them. A surgery colleague, Dr. Seth Newman, called from Haiti to describe to me a little Haitian girl who had been brought to him. He sent photos of her problem. Mirlande was born with a condition that occurs in approximately 1 of every 4,500 children: a congenital malformation of the digestive tract with a soft tissue tumor. In the U.S. this condition is routinely corrected at birth. In Haiti, no doctors had the expertise to perform the operation.

Seth and I conferred, and I told him, "Don't touch it. Don't do anything." It wasn't just that I had more expertise with this type of operation; Seth didn't have the resources or support to perform the surgery safely in Haiti. "She needs to come to the U.S.," I concluded.

Our hospital, Abington Memorial, coordinated the fundraising and logistics to get Mirlande and her father here, where Seth and I performed one of her operations. Ultimately I would perform six surgeries on Mirlande over the six months she lived in the United States. It was thrilling for all the staff involved with her transformation.

At home, Matt and I had our own scare: One of the boys suffered a seizure. I heard it through the baby monitor, a strange grinding noise that woke me, and when I got to the bedroom where the boys slept, he was in the midst of a full-on grand mal seizure. I started treatment and got him to the hospital. He made it through fine.

And I couldn't escape my own physical trials. I had two hernias repaired after my intense pregnancy with the twins. I suffered excessive fatigue from anemia and took iron infusions for months to boost my levels.

Through it all was the pressure—and blessing—of being a pediatric surgeon. And I was honored to be offered another appointment: as an attending surgeon at Children's Hospital of Philadelphia, perhaps the preeminent children's hospital in the world, certainly top five. That was worth a smile.

I sensed that I had reached a summit professionally, but that didn't mean I could stop growing and learning. I gained experience with every operation I performed, and that meant benefiting from outside advice, too. One day, the chair of my department at CHOP told me that I would have a better relationship with the nurse practitioners if I brought donuts for them now and then. At first, I was slightly offended; I had always had a good relationship with the NPs—anyway *I* thought so. Had someone said something?

"Some of them feel as if you hover," he said. "And micromanage."

Maybe I did. When I performed surgery at Abington, which was not a children's hospital—and certainly not one of the world's greatest, like CHOP—I got used to taking care of so many non-surgery tasks myself: wound check, post-op check, writing the prescription, discharging the patient. At CHOP, they had all the resources and nursing staff to support the surgeons, so all they really needed me to do was talk to the family before the operation, operate, then talk to the family after, then move on to the next patient.

I guess he was right. I couldn't have the nurses thinking I thought they weren't good at their job and resenting me. I needed to know they had my back.

"It's such an easy fix," my chairman advised.

I started bringing donuts.

Most of the operations I performed could be classified as routine, with almost zero risk of death or serious complication. But there were other, more intense and difficult challenges, the ones all those years of training were meant to prepare you for—though even all of that training might not be enough. A newborn arrived one day with a combination of Hirschsprung's disease, enterocolitis, and dead bowel, a complicated condition. The hand that the family had been dealt was tough enough without a very sick baby. The child went through multiple bouts of malabsorption and enterocolitis. I would care for him for years, pouring all I had into him with every procedure.

There was the mother of six who had parked her Chevy Suburban at the top of her driveway. Somehow it started to roll, running over her five-year-old son. He was pale when they brought him in. There was no blood return from the catheter I attempted to place in his subclavian vein. His organs were crushed. He bled to death internally in the trauma bay. It was devastating for all the staff. We weren't right for a while after that.

There were children who needed operations but who didn't have parents or guardians who loved them the way they deserved to be loved, or who outright abused them. In some of those cases, the children need surgery *because* of the abuse, like one case of "nonaccidental" trauma, though I never found out who beat up the two-year-old. When he was brought into Abington he was listless and soon lost consciousness. A head CT scan revealed a bleed on his brain. He needed an emergency craniotomy to drain the blood. For this surgery, I had help from a non-pediatric neurosurgeon; we were not at a children's hospital. The toddler weighed nine kilograms, and we had to calculate how much blood could be drained, how many platelets we would need, what size instruments to use, etc. Fortunately, one of my favorite pediatric anesthesiologists was available. You don't forget the details of such operations. Shaving the small head. Where exactly to make the burr hole in the skull. Knowing that, because it's a child's skull, you can't go too deep or you'll hit brain matter. We could see the epidural hematoma around the brain. The neurosurgeon and I couldn't have done the operation without each other.

After the surgery, the baby remained intubated and sedated in the recovery room. He was transferred to St. Christopher's because that was a children's hospital, and after several hours he was standing in his crib, hugging family, recognizing faces. The identity of the perpetrator was not evident; the child couldn't talk, and the other family members may not even have known what we discovered in the OR. Often it's only when you do scans and surgery that these horrors are discovered. After saving the child, you then do a skeletal survey—X-rays of all the bones of the child's or baby's body, looking for old healed fractures. The authorities start their investigation based on what they learn from us—how long ago this or that injury may have happened, so they can build a timeline of who was caring for the baby, when. It's almost never a random person. In nearly every case with a baby or two- or three-year-old, it's a family member with regular access.

Abusive households sometimes foster children. For those children, it's even more important for the surgeon to let the child know, through words and touch, how much they're valued, that it's going to be okay. When I'm in the OR with them, they are the most important person in the world. I always make sure they hear that and feel that. I feel the awesomeness of the responsibility, and the connection, too.

A fundamental principle of surgery: Control your emotions. In dealing with parents, for instance. At times I felt as if I entered into a near-meditative state before I spoke with them. If I didn't, and the situation was dire, then things would be even harder. If my patient was their third kid, for example, and the first two had already died (to take one particularly unfortunate case), then it was crucial for me not to betray panic or fully engage with the unfathomable terror and sadness they were feeling.

The calm extends to the OR, of course, no matter how complicated or routine the procedure. I did not play music all the time, though many surgeons do. As the surgeon, my mood dictates how the team functions. I can't be hyper or distant or it will put everyone else on edge. All is calm. *This is about to happen. Then this.* We all know there's going to be a lot of blood. I need you all ready with sponges to keep this under control. What if the baby's got a communicable disease? We're prepared. Everyone's double-gloved and masked.

If there is information that is vital to the care of this child, then of course I express it to the team in a measured manner. The best way to function competently is through utter calm and directness and thoroughness. If the operation turns crazy? I get even calmer. If things turn very dark, I must think only of the least bad outcome in the moment.

It had taken so much work and energy for me to become a pediatric surgeon. I had been through so much, not all of it welcome. A lot of it had built up scar tissue in me. Not all of those cracks in myself had been filled with gold epoxy.

Sometimes parents, seeing that I was the surgeon about to operate on their child, asked, "Where's the other doctor?" No, of course: It doesn't *have* to be a race thing. It doesn't *have* to be a gender thing. It doesn't have to be a race *and* gender thing. Parents react this way all the time when their child's surgeon is a stranger. It's normal. Parents want the doctor they know or the one they've heard about or who has been recommended. And there were many times that I was the recommended surgeon.

But other times it *is* a race thing. Once, while covering for another surgeon, I told a white couple that their child needed surgery. They said they would wait for the other doctor to return. I told them that that was too long; if they really wanted a surgeon other than me to operate, then they needed immediately to have their child transported to another hospital; there was still time for that. "Your little boy needs the operation soon," I said. "Or he's going to get sick and he could die. These are your options."

They asked if they could have a minute.

"Take the time you need," I said.

The mom got on the phone, walking halfway down the hall as she spoke. When she returned to me maybe five minutes later, she said, "Do we have a choice for doing the surgery?"

"No," I said. "So we're transferring him?"

"No. I talked to someone. They said you were qualified."

"Yes, I am," I said.

After their son's successful surgery, both mom and dad thanked me profusely. "He was so afraid," she said, "but my son said you held his hand and made him feel comfortable. And I want to thank you for that, too."

When I was younger such an episode would have upset me. I thought back to a moment earlier in my career when I entered the room in scrubs and the patient's family assumed I was there to empty the garbage or change the bedpan. I thought of occasions when I was passed over *even while wearing a white lab coat and a visible ID!*

"We're waiting for the doctor."

"I am the doctor."

"Oh . . . well, we're waiting for the head doctor."

But I had come to realize that people only know what they know. If you've only ever seen Black people cleaning the kitchen, cooking the food, driving the bus, then you don't know. And the idea of putting your child's very life in the hands of someone who looks different from everyone else you imagined capable of doing something like this—yeah, it's scary. Terrifying, actually. I understood that parents put a huge amount of trust in their pediatric surgeon. Yes, that's an understatement. It's a profound, emotional relationship. I wouldn't allow the instinctual reaction of one parent or one couple, white or not, to upset me. It's a privilege to be the one to repair a child, which is why I say to the parents, before I go into the OR, "I will take care of them like my own." Color shouldn't matter, right?

10

LEVELS OF CARE

When the paint on the walls in your medical facility is chipping, when the resources are inadequate, your patients feel bad about their surroundings and so do you. At St. Christopher's, one of the children's hospitals where I had privileges, I often feared my car would get broken into. I was all too familiar with that from working at Kings County in the 1990s. I was concerned about the proximity of the most recent shooting reported on the news, or the gunshots we actually heard. Patients and their families felt that, too. Upon entering the facility, it was clear our staff was overworked, often disgruntled. They lacked supplies. Many of our young patients lay in their rooms alone, no visitors, because one or both parents were working at jobs they couldn't leave even for a day, or because they had younger kids at home and no one to watch them.

I was also on staff at Children's Hospital of Philadelphia, CHOP, a sparkling facility in University City, the heart of West Philly. Most often each child had a parent in the room, or both. Many of the moms and dads had set up their "office" right there in the room, so they could work while being present with their sick or recovering child. For these parents, working remotely was no problem. If the parents couldn't be present, there was Child Life, hospital services designed to make the hospital experience more positive, with support animals, visiting celebrities, professional athletes, an outdoor courtyard.

Those amenities were rarely present at the other hospital.

Were the kids at the first hospital any less deserving of great health care than the kids at the second one?

Of course not. Insurance type, household income, and the color of your skin shouldn't matter, right?

My profession could be a lot physically, and emotionally and psychologically, too. I put so much of myself into every surgery, every child, that I probably needed a break, a chance to exhale for a moment or two. I was grateful that when I finished my days early, it allowed me to be with my own children while we were all still relatively alert, and I could read to them—*Goodnight Moon*, the Eric Carle books, children's books about their beautiful peach, caramel, and chocolate skin. On the other hand, because a surgeon's day so often begins before sunrise, I usually missed the kids' morning routine. That stung.

Dr. S. Allen Counter, the Harvard neurology professor I had heard speak at a Society of Black Academic Surgeons conference years earlier, knew a surgical mentor of mine, a staff surgeon at Mass General. Dr. Counter asked him if he knew of a doctor in Philadelphia to take care of a VIP patient. My former mentor called me. Would I be interested?

"I don't know what you mean by VIP," I said. "All my patients are VIPs." But sure, I said, happy to help. I was given an address, and a date and time to show up. It was the nicest house I'd ever seen on the Main Line, maybe anywhere. I waited quite a while in the anteroom before the VIP entered.

"How ya doin'?" said the famous actor. "Will Smith."

"I know who you are," I said.

To Philadelphians, Will is a favorite son going back to his rapper days with DJ Jazzy Jeff, then *The Fresh Prince of Bel-Air*. Even after he became a movie star and moved to L.A., he never forgot his roots.

Will told me that he would be in a remote area filming *After Earth*, and before he was on set for a considerable period of time, he wanted a physical exam, his eyes checked, and to see a dentist. It was pretty straightforward for me to set up; I arranged for visits to great doctors in each specialty, then compiled their reports and recommendations and guided him through the follow-up. I sent him a bill and that was that.

Sometime after that, at a book reading at the Temple Performing Arts Center, I recognized Will's father, Will Smith Sr. As I was leaving, I noticed Mr. Smith walking out, his breathing labored. I assisted him to his car. Days later I received a call from someone on his son's team asking if I would consider being his dad's "health care overseer." Among his father's major health problems, I learned, was recalcitrant heart failure.

I was not remotely interested in giving up pediatric surgery—not after all I'd been through to get there and what it meant to me—but the offer intrigued me. We settled on the title "health care consultant"; I would supervise his father's care at home, to start. Not long after, Will Sr.—who people called Daddio—suffered a health setback and needed briefly to be hospitalized, and after he was released I recommended he move to a facility. The facility chosen by his son happened to be just a couple miles from my home; I could easily check on Daddio during my commute to and from work. He was usually lively and happy to see me. He would let me know what was or was not working with the staff I'd placed around him. His heart was weak, but his mind and mouth were not. A veteran, he ran the ship; I was mostly just executing his wishes. As long as he had his oxygen tank and a continuous infusion of milrinone to keep his heart pumping, he would probably be all right. He would sometimes remove the oxygen when he went outside to smoke a cigarette (against his doctor's wishes).

On one visit, he and I sat talking by the garage while he smoked.

"You need to tighten this up," he said to me.

"What do you mean, 'tighten up'?"

"These nurses here. They're out of breath more than I am, and I'm on oxygen." We cracked up. Daddio took another puff to make his point. "The people you bring here are a reflection of you, and this is your business."

"What do you mean, 'This is my business'? I have a job. I get paid every two weeks. I'm a salaried surgeon. I'm looking after you because your son asked me to. This is not my main job."

He cocked his head. "Well, you need to think about it because you're doing a great job at it." That surprised me because he was always quick to point out little problems here and there.

He spent the next hour explaining the keys to owning and running a successful business. He had run a refrigeration and freezer business in West Philly, earning him the nickname "The Ice Man." Being a successful Black business owner in the 1950s and '60s was no easy feat, and I found myself taking notes as he spoke. It felt like I was sitting at my Uncle Frank's knee, soaking up any wisdom I could.

Our conversation awakened something in me. Was I an entrepreneur? Could I be? Wasn't it enough to be a doctor with a very special set of skills?

Soon enough, Will Jr. asked me to consult on other family members and friends—to offer second opinions, which often meant keeping them away from dubious procedures or unproven medications, and to provide a next level of care, something insurance would not cover. I wasn't going to be anyone's full-time doctor but I could provide guidance. Though I was not trained as a primary care physician, I had the expertise to listen to an account of symptoms, to diagnose, and to recommend next steps and specialists. I became the first call when serious health issues cropped up among any of Will's immediate or extended family or close friends. It was the kind of personalized health care that anyone would want.

•　•　•

A *Time* magazine article once noted the vitality of American presidents. In the previous half-century, it was reported, everyone who had held that position had lived to be at least eighty, and many much longer. One reason given was that they each had a single doctor dedicated to him while president and afterward, someone who knew their patient inside and out and wouldn't miss a thing. Jimmy Carter's family has a history of pancreatic cancer, which killed his father and three siblings; meanwhile, he was still going strong into his late nineties.

You can get really good care when your doctor really knows you.

Obviously, very few of us get treated like a current or former U.S. president. Most people, though, would like their doctor to be more available than your typical, stretched-thin primary care physician. It almost always takes money to get that kind of care. If you have it, you might opt for a relatively new model called "concierge medicine," a method of primary care medicine that gives the patient a more customized, regular relationship with his or her doctor, in exchange for a membership fee.

I started a concierge medicine practice.

Like most Americans, I assumed that millionaires and society's top earners had the best of everything, including medical care.

Not true. Not even when you're rich. Despite their affluence, my patients, in past and sometimes current health care situations, were often assessed first by the color of their skin. Simply being Black means often getting less respect, less attention, less care—and having poorer health outcomes—regardless of income status. The determining condition isn't being Black *and* poor. It isn't being Black and uneducated. It's being Black, period.

Having taken care of several Black multimillionaires, I'm quite sure that had I not been present when it was time for them to have their procedure, things might have gone differently. Had I not been advising some of my patients, they might not have been offered more than one treatment option, including a less invasive one. In short, they would have been treated like everybody else who looks like them.

How can I possibly know this? I've seen it too many times. An African American singer whose tour was interrupted by a syncopal episode (fancy term for fainting) reached out, worried. He was thousands of miles from home, and I sent him—an educated, affluent, insured Black man—to a hospital near his location. I had called ahead and provided the hospital with both an account of what happened and my patient's medical history. The supervisor assured me the patient would be cared for and that the doctor would give me a call after the evaluation. A bit later I received a call from the singer's manager.

"How'd it go?" I asked.

"We're in the hospital parking lot. They discharged him. Said nothing's wrong and to follow up when we get back home."

What? He was sent away untreated and, it would turn out, unexamined. I called the hospital and lit into them about not taking my patient's condition seriously. They should have done an EKG on his heart, done labs, *at least checked his vitals*! They had promised to do all of it when we spoke—and then they saw his face. Numerous Black patients of mine, also out of town, experienced the same indifference and irresponsible (non-) health care.

A California study showed that babies born to the richest Black mothers are more likely to die than babies born to the poorest white mothers.[1] The same is true of the mothers. How is that possible? Because the racism at the root is still a factor.

Over 90 percent of my concierge clientele is Black. My patients are often more than just successful in their field and wealthy: They're also role models. They're not just helping to provide dedicated health care to their immediate and extended families but giving to their communities. I see my role as helping them to continue to influence and bring joy to others. If that brilliant, innovative chief executive or lawyer or former NFL star drops dead of a heart attack at forty-two, they leave behind their family and all the others who depended on them. But they leave another void. They are no longer there as a needed role model. No longer there to do the kind of philanthropy and community outreach that, in real dollars, is far less common in Black communities, despite the need generally being far greater. In each case, I honestly feel as if I'm providing medical advice for more than that one, privileged patient. That person is responsible for many people's lives and livelihoods, while I'm responsible for keeping him or her healthy. So, yeah, maybe a little like the president's personal physician.

As a concierge doctor or health care consultant, I also serve as a repository for my patients' medical records as they travel the world. It keeps me on my toes, creating ways for them to receive needed health care whether they're out on the road or at home. (I am required to be medically licensed in each state where my patients reside.) Because my patients value my services, some of which are not reimbursable by insurance, compensation is commensurate with the value they place on it. This allows me to continue to care for those who can't afford to pay or who are ineligible for health insurance, by often waiving my fees for consultation and surgery.

I provide equally good, dedicated care to all my patients, of course, regardless of how much they're paying me, even as the rich ones are helping to subsidize the not-so-rich ones.

On top of the concierge practice and my own pediatric surgery practice I opened near home, I was still also performing surgeries at two hospitals two days a week. I needed to find a way to be more with *my* own—my young kids—before it was too late.

11

OUTCOMES I DIDN'T COUNT ON

As a Black doctor, a woman doctor, a surgeon, I felt I needed to do more than my day job: I had an obligation to the community to give back. *To whom much is given, much is required.*

A mantra in the Black community, from the New Testament, Luke 12:48. I had a responsibility to let others, especially kids and teens and younger people, see me and talk to me and know what was possible. Because I was involved in the care of a number of prominent folks and they liked me, I started to receive invitations to high-profile occasions. Months before, I had been invited to attend a Barack Obama event for his second term in office. Matthew and I had attended the first inauguration four years earlier, on our own, in the freezing cold for twelve hours. He understood the importance of being there with me at the Capitol.

But Matthew was growing impatient with the increasing demands on my time. Being a pediatric surgeon was consuming enough. I felt he struggled to understand why I seemed compelled also to take on this whole new concierge medicine practice and all the extra work that came with it. We weren't broke—a working surgeon and a working dentist, after all. I was using my hands and my brain to help children and babies in need—did I have to be so involved in *other* causes, too? Inspiring young people: good, fine, but those weren't my children. He believed that when I wasn't doing surgery, my responsibility was at home, as a mother and a wife—honestly, not an unreasonable request. His ideal weekend, especially when I was not on call, was one where we parked our car on Friday after work and didn't move it again until Monday morning. That didn't sound awful, especially after the stresses of the week, and I certainly wanted time with our three sons—but I also wanted to own a business, to encourage the next generation, and for Matt to take the ride with me.

He was not interested. I made my case, arguing that when you give back you get back, that concierge medicine would boost our income, that a win for me was a win for us, and why don't you join me at the movie premiere? It was not the life he wanted nor the one he had signed up for. Our different views of my personal and professional growth and our family were taking a toll.

I thought I might just be done with the physical trauma to my body— I'd been through laparoscopy, days of labor, two Cesarean sections, uterine biopsies, egg retrievals, fertility treatments, miscarriage, two hernia operations—but in 2013 I had my most significant medical challenge yet.

For years I had vowed that someday I would do the Broad Street Run, ten miles down one of Philadelphia's most famous thoroughfares, and in May, after months of training and in the best shape of my adult life, I completed it. Exactly one month after I crossed the finish line, I found myself on the verge of death.

I had had uterine bleeding for nearly a year, which I'd initially thought was just a heavy menstrual cycle after my twins. A uterine biopsy ruled out cancer. I scheduled an endometrial ablation, which is usually a simple, same-day procedure to burn the uterine lining and halt the bleeding.

As a surgeon, I should know not to use the phrase "simple procedure" to describe anything.

My surgery was set for a Friday, a potential red flag (if your surgeon's on call for the weekend, great; if your surgeon's heading out of town for the weekend and something goes wrong post-op, not so great). Then my start time was delayed for hours, another red flag (fewer staff around on weekends generally, so the later the start time, the less staff available), which should have been my cue to reschedule. I did not. In my pre-op appointment, I should have pointed out to the surgeon that I might not be a good candidate for this procedure given my history of prior operations on my uterus and the weakened tissue that resulted. I did not. I decided to be a patient. I ignored my own doctorly instincts.

After the procedure, the surgeon headed out of town. I was released from the hospital. Later that afternoon I went to the mall. I was looking forward to the following morning, when Matthew and I planned to take the boys to Sesame Place. But very late that night, I awoke with chills—and I'm so glad I did because waking up saved my life.

I was septic. Sepsis often kills people in their sleep, as bacteria spreads through their bloodstream. My condition steadily deteriorated; the expression "circling the drain" came to me. My neighbor Jane, an NICU nurse who had just finished a night shift, drove me to the ER in the early morning, while Matthew stayed back with the boys. I walked into the hospital unassisted, but when I saw my vital signs, my subsequent labs, and then started vomiting bile, I knew I was in big trouble. Soon, I couldn't walk at all. I became completely disoriented. I felt close to the worst I'd physically ever felt in my life. I surrendered to unconsciousness. I don't know what happened next, of course, but I'm told that the doctors resuscitated me through the day and following night, keeping me alive. I knew them all. I woke up with a catheter in my bladder that I had no recollection of when it was placed.

Before I was wheeled into the OR for my follow-up surgery—an emergency hysterectomy and salpingectomy, needed to address the complications caused by the first surgery—I remember Robeson asking the doctors, "Where are you taking my mommy?"

In my room there were six doctors and staff standing around my bed, never a good sign. The surgeon scheduled to perform the procedures was gifted technically and had a terrific bedside manner. He told me we had to do it *now*. The senior assisting resident was my former medical student; two years earlier I had operated on her son. Another surgeon was a friend; during the NFL season he and I talked football every Monday about our favorite team, the Eagles. I could tell from looking at his face that this was serious. There were no smiles. I was critically ill. Surgeons know when you've got one foot in the grave.

During the operation, a perforation was found in my uterus. It had been created from the procedure two days prior, when the ablation tools that were supposed to burn only the lining of my uterus instead burned through its full thickness, allowing dead uterine tissue, along with normal flora, to spread into my abdominal cavity and throughout my body. ("Normal flora" is bacteria in your body that's fine so long as it stays where it needs to circulate.)

Without that trip back to the OR, I would have died. It was a good thing I entered the hospital in the best shape of my life from training for the Broad Street Run. That might have saved me, too. In the ICU, I lost half of my circulating blood volume. I did not want them to give me a blood transfusion unless it was once again a matter of life or death. My hemoglobin level had gone from 14 to 7, just on the edge.

After being a doctor for more than a decade and a half, the entire experience as patient, with its repeated but unpredictable ups and downs, taught me that the physical healing of the tissue, the muscle, the forming and hardening of the scar: All of that is the easier healing. And it happens first. The emotional and spiritual healing take much longer. Such an experience changes you profoundly. You have to allow yourself to feel the uncomfortableness of the situation, to be sad, to be pissed, to be kind to yourself. If you're the caregiver for someone going through this, you have to be patient and supportive with your loved one, because yes, while in six to eight weeks their flesh will be strong, it may take much longer for them to heal mentally and emotionally. For everyone in the world who has been through a similar surgical odyssey, a botched operation, an unplanned operation, maybe one for cancer or another life-threatening condition, the experience turns your world upside down, and it stays that way long after the procedure is technically complete.

I felt another transformation. Had I not been ill, septic, and dying, I would not know and see God the way I did afterward. My health, the operation that caused the complication, feeling at my lowest point, my weakest and most physically downtrodden, nearly losing my life, the emergency follow-up that saved my life, being a patient in the ICU, searching for a seed of faith: From that whole experience I emerged stronger than I had ever felt. I had a fearlessness, except the fear of God. I was determined to live a life of no regret.

I knew how fortunate I was to have survived sepsis. I appreciated everything in a new light. I remember how quiet my hospital room felt, and how thrilled I was after being discharged to turn on a radio and hear music. With renewed gratitude, I saw and felt everything in my life that I might previously have taken for granted. But not everything was a source of uplift. At home, recovering, whenever Matthew and I started a conversation, it quickly devolved into an argument. I couldn't help but think: *God didn't spare my life for this.*

There were other things I could no longer go back to—specifically, the pediatric surgery division of my hospital, Abington. I had been their main pediatric surgeon, and while I was incapacitated by my surgeries, they were forced to shut down for lack of coverage. They had to refer my patients to the nearby children's hospitals. I was not seeing patients, not operating, and thus generating no revenue for the hospital. And though the general surgery division remained vibrant, general surgeons cannot operate on newborn babies. When I was ready to operate again, I would have to search for a new pediatric surgery job, perhaps even in another state.

I felt more committed than ever to help find solutions to problems in my community that went beyond health care. I had created a non-profit, It Takes Philly, Inc. (a play on "It takes a village"), to help expose underserved youth to professionals and offer these young people direct contact and feedback about goal-setting, self-esteem, and delayed gratification. I galvanized my successful friends to participate and share insights into how they had gotten where they were. We could nurture in these kids the idea that if they feel responsible for their success in life, they'd be more likely to succeed, professionally and personally. I wanted to add structure to what was provided to me through the African Free school, exposure to a Black woman physician, visits to college campuses, and more. It Takes Philly did that.

I also had the opportunity to coauthor a paper that examined a question that had increasingly interested and bothered me for years: Do children of color truly have worse health outcomes after certain surgeries than white children, all else being equal? That is, when there is no difference in the level of comorbidity, and no difference in the facilities where the surgeries are being performed, and the procedure is the same, can you discern a disparity? And if so, why?

While on staff at CHOP and working with their Policy Lab, which did community-engaged research, I looked through charts of patients to see which procedure would make for the most effective comparison. I landed on the congenital condition called malrotation and midgut volvulus, in which the intestine, instead of being anchored by ligaments to the back wall of the abdominal cavity, is untethered, allowing it to twist on itself, which can choke its blood supply. If you don't operate immediately, the intestine can die, and the child can die. Our hospital had done many such procedures on children aged five and under. We looked at outcomes, as well as how much time elapsed between the child's arrival at the hospital, when their condition was diagnosed, and when the operation began.

By removing the variable of *pre*-hospital care, we established a much more controlled environment. Had we measured pre-hospital care—something very tough to calculate, like "time from symptom onset to arrival at ER"—it would have made comparisons among patients more difficult. Such variables matter, no question. For instance, a child with midgut volvulus whose parents don't have a car, or who don't have money for a car service, even in such an emergency, might well have a worse surgical outcome because it took longer to get her to the hospital. (Remember my mother, when she went into labor with me, taking the Broad Street subway to the hospital because no taxi was going to pick her up?) A child who lives far from a better-resourced hospital (with pediatric subspecialists in surgery, radiology, critical care, etc.) would take longer to get there, regardless of whether they traveled by car or mass transit, than a child who lived in the neighborhood. A child whose parents are not citizens might hesitate to go to a hospital—even in the midst of a terrible health emergency—because they fear deportation or arrest and an even worse outcome. These factors matter, of course, but we wanted to set them aside and see what we found if we "started the clock" at the time the newborn or child showed up at the medical facility.

We found that it took longer for Hispanic patients to get diagnosed and then operated on, and had poorer health outcomes, than white or Black children; while Black children had worse outcomes than white children, the statistically significant disparity was between Hispanic and non-Hispanic. Hispanic children had the highest incidence of profound disease (needed more bowel removed) and the highest percentage of death from this condition.

The results were startling—and, for some, simply too much to accept.

The paper we produced was titled, "Hispanic Disadvantage in the Surgical Outcomes of Malrotation and Midgut Volvulus," and it was published in the *Journal of the American College of Surgeons*. I presented our findings at the American Academy of Pediatrics. I presented them at the American College of Surgeons. And I presented them at CHOP, one of the hospitals I was affiliated with. When I concluded the presentation, one faculty member said, "That's not true."

As wrong and arrogant as he was, his reaction was understandable. Most doctors, which of course includes most pediatric surgeons, take care of children regardless of who they are and where they're from—or at least they intend to. They're children! How can you be biased? For the vast majority of us doctors, there is no Black, white, brown, rich, poor: We take care of everyone the same—right? So it's hard to swallow statistically significant data showing that—all else being equal—children of color may have poorer health outcomes. It can't be true!

But it was. Fortunately, I was prepared for such pushback. I pointed out that we had done this study in conjunction with the Policy Lab, known for its meticulous research. Their staff helped us to analyze the data we had gathered. And a senior researcher of the Policy Lab, an author on my paper, was there at the presentation, and she stood up for the work, literally. "It *is* true," she countered. The on-staff pediatricians and statisticians who had reviewed and worked on the research also backed up our results.

The doctor who disagreed attributed the worse outcomes for Hispanic children to the fact that it took patients of color longer to be brought to the hospital, arguing that if more time had passed "until we touch them, then they're going to have a poorer outcome." It would have been a valid critique . . . except we specifically excluded that variable! So what explains that *once a brown child was in our hospital, he or she waited longer to get to the OR than a white child?*

Perhaps it's "the squeaky wheel gets the grease": white families more frequently knowing what to ask for, and being more comfortable asking for it; perhaps Hispanic families feel less comfortable saying something on the order of, "Where's the attending surgeon? We need a doctor right now!" It could also be a cultural thing. For many, there may be a language barrier, and it may take time to find a translator—especially if the better-resourced hospitals are in neighborhoods with fewer Spanish-speaking community members. In fact, we dug deeper and found that Hispanic patients treated at a hospital that served more Hispanic patients had better outcomes and fewer bowel resections.

And that was that.

I don't mean by those four words that we had settled the issue. I'm afraid I mean it more negatively. I mean that our results just got ignored. *And that was that.* Like so many conversations then and in the past about racial and ethnic disparities in health outcomes, people weren't listening, or believing, or doing all that much about it, including many in the health care field who had surely witnessed these disparities themselves. When presenting the findings at my own hospital, I got looks that can only be described as *How dare you?* As if we had set out to point fingers at our own. Many of the people at our presentations were just not ready for what we had concluded, never mind that our study examined more than 4,200 patient results, that it went through peer review, and that it had been published in a scholarly journal that they respected.

The point was not to disparage my hospital, an incredible institution. Evidence of racial inequity and outcome disparity in health care is not exactly hard to find at any hospital. Yet many doctors and authorities in hospitals and health care settings around the country, as well as lawmakers and regular citizens, were—are—unwilling to do anything about a problem that damages us all. Many simply couldn't—and still can't—accept the fact that continuing racial bias is the problem. Like my colleague, many people in health care and outside it take issue with such findings, insisting they're the result of problems with the methodology. Or that patients of color simply start off less healthy. Or don't properly take care of themselves. Or some other garbage.

Maybe the most obstructive problem to "solving" systemic racism is that many people refuse to believe it exists. They get defensive if you tell them that it does, even when you provide proof. They don't like it because it means it's been happening on their watch; they're doctors, after all, driven by science and logic, and the findings seem to implicate their involvement, or at least inaction, regarding this problem. They're dead certain that the problem you're pointing to cannot have causes in continued neglect, selfishness, or outright prejudice.

It's got to be something else. It's always something else.

What do we do, then, with evidence, such as that laid out in a study published in *Pediatrics* in mid-2020 that showed that apparently healthy African American children were three and a half times likelier than their white counterparts to die within thirty days after surgery?[1] Could it mean that *race itself is a risk factor*?

Yes. Race is a risk factor. Can we please stop blaming the patient?

My increased professional commitments and activism came at a steep personal cost.

Increasingly, I was finding my voice, a public voice. I wanted to use it to help directly the people I'd grown up with, the ones who hadn't been able to rise above, for one reason or a hundred reasons. I wanted to embrace my mother's and my family's heritage of advocacy and activism, all those lessons of my youth: *Each one, teach one ... Lift as you climb ... He ain't heavy, he's my brother.* Those lessons had nourished and supported me throughout my childhood and adolescence and young adulthood, and through all those difficult years struggling to become a doctor. I felt as if I was on increasingly solid footing, and I wanted to use my strength to help lift up others, however I could.

I was coming into my own and embracing my gifts. I was no longer the same person my husband had married. There was a cultural disconnect that he did not understand or, I felt, want to accept. Matthew and I had fallen in love while we were both residents at Pitt—and yet, tough as that environment was, it was not the real world. We were in the real world now, and had been through a lot, and I was changing. Near-death can do that to you.

I felt there was a greater purpose for me. And I wouldn't let anything hold me back from discovering it.

Early in 2014, I filed for divorce.

I don't regret the marriage. Without it, we would not have our three magnificent children, each a combination of Matthew and me and also completely and beautifully their own person.

Together we had joined Salem Baptist Church in Abington, not far from where we lived, and I took even greater solace now in the congregation. During the divorce proceedings (which I kept quiet about), I couldn't help but think of all the things I had done "wrong" during the marriage. And I was still not fully recovered from my emergency surgery, though it had happened many months before. But I always left Bible study feeling hopeful. In the stories, I found parallels to my own life, and they gave me comfort, reminding me that whatever I was feeling was okay because things were going to turn out all right. I was heartened being around the older women, all of whom had endured heartache and disappointment of so many kinds, yet carried on with grace. They, too, showed me that it would be okay.

There are few things more powerful than praying women, mothers and grandmothers of the church, and on those days my heart was particularly heavy, the women embraced me and prayed for me. They refueled me, validated me, helped me restore my sense of worth. It was also a way to get out of the house for ninety minutes and have some time away, because though Matthew and I were separated, we still lived under the same roof.

I had been interviewing for pediatric surgery positions, a far less fraught process this time around, now that I had been doing it for years and had developed a positive reputation. Still, I couldn't expect to find something wherever I chose. I had privileges at CHOP and St. Christopher's, but Abington, my home institution, had paid my salary. I was offered a job in Charlotte, North Carolina.

New legal arrangements designated Pennsylvania the kids' home, foreclosing the possibility of me bringing them with me; the judge ruled that the boys would stay in the Philadelphia area for the school year and come to North Carolina for the summer. Weekends throughout the year would alternate, which would be complicated, expensive, and stressful. I got up to Philly as often as I could, but it was more or less an atrocious time down in Charlotte for me, in a five-thousand-square-foot home, mostly alone, missing my children horribly, basically just commuting during the workweek between hospital and home, where I went right to bed.

But the rare luxury of time alone also allowed me to reflect on important things I'd mostly avoided. Since graduating from high school, I'd been through so many years of college, medical school, medical training, and medical practice, all the while experiencing significant adversity, overt and covert racism, sexism, gaslighting, character assassination, unfounded criticism of my performance—and I was still standing. How? I could just as easily have succumbed to any one or two of those challenges. I had always been interested in equality and equity, in opportunities versus outcomes. I wondered why some of us land on our feet and some don't. How come I was in the first group?

THE ONES NOT SUPPOSED
TO MAKE IT

Rev. Marshall Mitchell, pastor of Salem Baptist, had been asking me for months if I would give a sermon, and for months I had turned him down. I was deeply honored by the request, but I didn't feel as if I had something to say. Perhaps one day.

Though I was now shuttling between states, I always tried to make Bible study because of the people there, especially two older women, Carole and Malessia. I felt comfortable enough to confide in them that I had recently filed for divorce—something that until then I had shared only with my pastor and closest family and friends. I opened up about how challenging it was to be starting a new life as a single parent to three young children, but I believed I had made the right choice— never mind the demands of pediatric surgery.

On Mother's Day after church, a handsome man walked up to me. I recalled having seen him in church some months before, sitting with two children—a teen girl and boy. We had shared a few words then.

Now he said to me, "How you doin'? I know we haven't talked

much since we saw each other some time ago. But I heard you got a new job. Congratulations! And that you're single."

Wait—where did he learn all that?

The man must have read my confused expression because he nodded toward someone in the crowd nearby. Carole.

"My mom," he said.

Soon after that I said yes to a date with him—Byron Drayton—even though I was out of town far more than I was in Philly. He was an entrepreneur with a couple of businesses going, and he also worked as a controller for an accounting firm in Washington, D.C., so he spent most of his workdays out of town, too.

And I said yes, too, to Reverend Mitchell's invitation to speak. I realized I *did* have something to say.

The second Sunday of June 2014, Pentecost Sunday, was almost exactly a year since I had almost died from sepsis. I know I am always at the mercy of God, but on that day in 2013 I had felt it more acutely than ever. And now, twelve months later, I was taking the pulpit at Salem Baptist Church.

I'm no preacher, obviously, but in the weeks leading up to the day, I thought often of Uncle Frank and the hours I had spent sitting outside his book-filled study while he was in there crafting his sermons. I thought of his booming voice, every sentence wise and deep and full of faith and love of God. It took me a while to bring together my own thoughts and find the relevant Bible verses, then to write it all down. If the sermon was to mean something, I needed to examine and be open about *everything*. How had I survived it all? How had I ended up in that place, in front of all those parishioners and friends, giving a sermon, telling the congregation a story that might be full of wisdom for them? I wanted to impart a positive message and talk about how, when I got to where I had wanted to be for so long, it really *did* feel as if a huge burden was lifted from my shoulders. Maybe it was going through my divorce proceedings that allowed that realization to filter down—yet another tough challenge faced, and look at me, still standing. Something had fallen into place.

I didn't know that anyone who had ever been up on that pulpit had spoken more candidly but I said what I thought needed saying.

My message on this day was especially important for younger people to hear. For anyone who had been through something like I had. I treated newborns and babies and children in my operating room as if they were my own, and now I wanted to treat the young people in the pews as if they were my own, too.

"A Demonstration of the Spirit's Power"

ALA STANFORD

Sunday, June 8, 2014, 10 a.m.
Salem Baptist Church

"Thank you, Pastor Mitchell, Salem family, my friends, family, acquaintances, colleagues, and my sons," I addressed the congregation. "Thank you so much for taking time out of your Sunday to share it with me.

"Recently, while I was on a plane coming back to Philly, I was flipping through my Bible for something that might motivate me to write. At first I found nothing. And then I landed at First Corinthians 2nd chapter, and I said, 'My *God*, this is exactly the message to share.' Paul is speaking in the church to the people of Corinth. He knows there is strife among them. Many are more interested in the wisdom of man and worldly things than in the wisdom of God. Paul shares a testimony to what God can do and how He can move in your life through the Holy Spirit.

"I am a woman, some might even say a successful woman, but I have had my share of challenges, disappointments, and despair. But for God's grace and mercy I would not be here before you. As a child, it was hard to understand who and what the Holy Spirit was. Perhaps for some adults, too. For me it's something you feel. It's how God speaks to you. It's how things unfold and problems are solved and you have strength to keep going, providing finances when you know they had run out, but the Holy Spirit made the way out of no way. But there are impediments and obstacles to feeling the Holy Spirit in your life. Sometimes you can hurt. Sometimes you can hurt so bad that you don't have the energy to pray. You are so despondent, down, and depressed that *that* becomes the main spirit that fills your mind.

"We lost a great woman recently who shared her story with us in her book *I Know Why the Caged Bird Sings*. With her manifesto, Dr. Maya Angelou gave a voice to many abused girls and boys. She gave a voice to me. Abuse, whether it's verbal, physical, or sexual abuse, will cause you shame, embarrassment, loneliness, hurt, confusion. It robs you of your self-esteem and your womanhood or your manhood before you have a chance to know what being a woman or a man is. You become unsure, introverted.

"You're afraid to talk about it. You embody the hurt. This turmoil can distance you from the Holy Spirit. It may cause you to settle in your life because you are afraid something better won't come along. You ask yourself, who would love me, right? You are used to people taking what they want from you. You fear you aren't good enough. We are worth exactly what we want in life, but you have to believe it or you won't attract something better. We have to teach our young girls and women: You are a *Queen*. We have to teach our young boys and men: You are a *King*. Take a moment to realize your worth and what you deserve. You are God's child. Some of these experiences of abuse prevent us from knowing our worth, create doubt, chaos, and disbelief of our God-given abilities and talents. Only God could take a Black girl born in North Philly, child of a teenage mother, born impoverished, abused, with average grades, and give her an unshakable spirit to persevere, make her a pediatric surgeon. Only the Holy Spirit has the power to do that.

"You might think, 'Oh, He made you a doctor.' No, no, no. It goes much deeper, much more profound than that. Through my giving to others, He provided a vehicle that I could use to love and protect His children and take the energy and the shame from a negative experience and transform it, allowing children to feel love and confidence in a safe environment. And I, at the same time, get to do my part to help recognize when a child has experienced what I did, and not have her or him ever feel so alone.

"Dr. Angelou speaks about the Caged Bird, who feels imprisoned in the narrow cage of bars, with her wings clipped and feet tied, so she opens her throat to sing. And here I am. From my pain comes power. From those terrible experiences I found my gift and purpose. It's funny how you don't realize as a child that things are a challenge or a struggle until someone mentions that you are broke. I didn't know to be unhappy. We were happy and broke, eating peanut butter sandwiches, hot dogs and baked beans, and grilled cheese sandwiches made underneath the oven in the broiler, the cheese so thick you wanted the bubble but you didn't want it to burn. In the winter, when we didn't have heat, we took turns ironing the sheets in our beds, so we would be warm. My brother and I had each other. Being broke doesn't keep you from dreaming. Being broke doesn't keep you from having a desire for something better for you and your family. We were the ones not supposed to make it, on public assistance, with teenage parents, with high school counselors telling us 'College is not for you.' The world had *low* or *no* expectations for us. But that didn't matter to us. Overt racism. Covert racism. Being the ones left behind and forgotten. Because as I marched on, thinking I was in control, God had a different plan. Despite being in a home where we lived paycheck to paycheck, where we took SEPTA to get where we needed to go, we made it to college and professional school. We didn't have money but we had *love*. We had the power of God.

"Abuse happens to all kinds of young girls, short and tall, fat and skinny, light-skinned and dark-skinned, short hair, no hair, bought hair, to those from single-parent homes and where both parents are at home. Those hurt or abused by someone who was supposed to love and protect them can be scarred for life. The same is true for our young men. Our childhood is the most malleable, constructive time in our lives. Abuse causes young men and women to think less of themselves, to expect less from others, to keep them from tapping into their true potential, their God-given gifts. It creates so much clutter and chaos in their minds that when God speaks, they can't hear His voice. They can't hear Him helping to create paths and opportunities and order to their steps. All those eighteen years old and under, please stand."

Thunder of feet shuffling. The children in the church stood. I hadn't realized until then just how many young people were in attendance. I addressed the seated congregation: "When you see a young child or a young adult, tell them, 'You are smart, you are beautiful, can I give you a hug?' Tell them, 'I love your smile.' They may not believe it that day, but if you say it to them often enough, eventually they will believe it, and you will empower them! I, Ala Stanford, did not come to you as a preacher, nor someone with great eloquence and wisdom. I came only proclaiming a testimony about God and a demonstration of the Spirit's power. Yes, we were poor and succeeded. But many of us have that story. With my 'success,' I continue to strive toward significance. We should all pray and thank God for our blessings. But more significant is that we are a blessing to someone else."

It's amazing for me to read those words now and see where my mind was. That was an awakening. Everything raw and open. An epiphany about my abuse and how the pain and my eventual wisdom about it intersected with everything else, including my success. That sermon was like a letter to God that I was blessed enough to be sharing with others.

Bring it on. I got this.

That was my approach to whatever came my way next. I had been bruised, but I wasn't battered. Belief in myself and faith in God would sustain me—the former, practically and physically, the latter, mentally and spiritually. I didn't need signs, but whatever He had in store for me, I was ready for the challenge.

And challenges came, as they always do.

The November after my sermon, while I was working in North Carolina, one of my sons had a medical emergency at school. I felt it would have been managed differently, better, if I had been present. Matt got him to the hospital as soon as he was called, but I heard it took a while before anyone at the school had thought to bring down the fever with Tylenol, a cool cloth, and some ice. Had they forgotten the entire play-by-play I'd given them? And the Tylenol with his name on it?

I hopped on a plane and went to my children. I did not finish my clinic in Charlotte. I told them I had to go, jumped in my car, and sped off to the airport in my scrubs. When I arrived back north, the boys were all happy to see me. I slept on the couch in their room. My son was okay, but I felt a sense of helplessness. I was determined to get back to Philly for good as soon as possible. This wasn't working. When I told my mom, she pointed out that I was employed in North Carolina. "You can't come home without a job," she said.

"I'm going home to my kids. I don't care if I have to work at Starbucks. I'm getting out of here."

I gave notice to the hospital in Charlotte. I had to return the bonus and pay back the relocation fee. But by April of 2015, I was back in Philadelphia with my children. The judge immediately changed the custody arrangements to equal sharing. I found a two-bedroom apartment, barely a thousand square feet. It was humbling but it was all I could afford; I was paying my mortgage in Charlotte, the marital home mortgage, student loans, day care services, and car note, all while suddenly receiving no income. I depleted my savings and maxed out my credit cards. My credit score was shit—400! I was fortunate that the application for the apartment complex had been approved in December, right after my son's seizure and before my credit tanked with all this debt and no income.

I landed a pediatric surgical position at Cooper University Health

Care and Cooper Medical School of Rowan University, and was hired to be on the faculty of two departments there, Surgery and Pediatrics. The move back north also meant I could see more of Byron, who had three kids himself—Byron Jr., Myles, and Maya—all older than mine.

It would be a couple months before I started at Cooper, which was a very good thing, because now I needed surgery on another part of my body, the lifeblood (aside from the brain) for a surgeon.

My hands.

I had come to feel increasingly compromised by the very tools that God had given me to do what I do. My hands are not dainty. They're size seven and strong but very gentle. But the wear and tear of performing thousands of surgeries was finally catching up with me: I was suffering regular shooting pain. Even a young surgeon's hands, wrists, and arms will feel fatigued after a six-, eight-, or ten-hour surgery day, but they'd never notice it during: We're so focused on the patient and the job before us that we don't think of it; we're not even a person in those moments, but a vessel with a mission.

Over time, I began to take more explicit care of my hands, especially my wrists. On my commute to work I sometimes wore an ACE wrap—the kind you put your thumb through, that you can buy at CVS or Walgreens. Now and then I took ibuprofen for the pain.

Things never got so bad that instruments were falling out of my hands. But it was painful to open a jar. In the shower I could barely wash my body. On the drive between Charlotte and Philadelphia, with my hands fastened to the steering wheel for eight hours, I could feel it in my wrists. Around Thanksgiving we were all at Carole's (or "Byron's mom's," as she was increasingly known to me) watching an awards show, and when I snapped my fingers, I felt a spark down my wrist. Nerve compression.

It's not unusual for surgeons to require carpal tunnel surgery; for those of us who operate on small children, it's even more likely. (We're also prime candidates for cervical neck surgery, because we spend hours and hours standing while facing down, and the head is quite heavy.)

Now I had pain in both wrists, bilaterally—inside and outside the wrists. It wasn't excruciating, but it was consistent and debilitating, and I began to wonder if I had performed my last operation.

Once again, I found myself in the OR as a patient.

The procedure was successful, thank God. And I had time to heal and do physical therapy. In the interim, I agreed to accompany Daddio—Will Smith's dad—to a doctor's appointment one day. I couldn't drive yet, so he offered to pick me up. Right away his gaze went to my bandaged-up wrists.

"What the hell did you do!" he asked.

"It's not what you think!" I said, and we both laughed.

In the period before my appointment at Cooper began, I kept busy. I hate sitting around, so besides PT and spending as much time as possible with my boys, I involved myself with lots of organizations, as I always had—the Society of Black Academic Surgeons (SBAS), Alpha Kappa Alpha Sorority, the Philadelphia Academy of Surgery, and others. Often I volunteered ("Front Row" Ala) to help with event planning, such as a big splash for the SBAS at the Four Seasons.

One fall day in 2015, just months after I'd started my new gig at Cooper, I watched on TV as Pope Francis, visiting America, delivered a homily at St. Patrick's Cathedral in Manhattan. It was translated into English. At one point, he apologized for the abuse that had happened in the Church.

Before that moment, I had never heard someone in a position of authority say those simple words. *I'm sorry.* In a sense, it felt a little as if *he* was apologizing to *me*, even though the Church had not been the source of my abuse. It nearly knocked me over. My faith is strong; it was as if God was saying the words through Pope Francis.

I'm sorry. It was not your fault.

I don't know that it meant anything that sometime after that, following a Sunday church service, I was running an errand in my car when a drunk driver rear-ended me, tearing my left shoulder, again jeopardizing my surgical career. I did physical therapy, acupuncture—nothing worked. I had surgery on my shoulder. Once more I wondered if I would ever again be able to operate.

Did God have another plan for me?

13

WHAT DO YOU WANT TO BE?

Church members and friends often inquired, "How's that Haitian child with the tumor you operated on? Have any new pictures?"

Salem Baptist Church, led by Pastor Mitchell, had done mission trips to Haiti—traditional missions where you bring food, clothes, shoes, flip-flops, talk about Christianity, that sort of thing. But now he asked me, "What do you think about building a hospital in Haiti? And bringing medical care down there?"

I knew I wanted to do more than what I was doing within the walls of my hospitals and private practice. "I don't know about a hospital," I said, "but I can certainly provide medical care."

In November of 2015, we went down there—nurses, physician assistants, pharmacists—and nonmedical people, too—an insurance claims adjuster, a videographer. The pastor, me, and my father, now retired, who knew nothing about medicine but wanted to join because he felt he had more to give.

In Port-au-Prince and the area outside it, I saw all the different things that can happen to people without basic preventive medical care. Yes, it was so incredibly poor, but Haiti can feel like a paradox.

Children without clothes on the lower half of their bodies. Young girls in the wee hours of the morning with buckets on their heads to get to a stream to bathe themselves before work and school. Kids running toward you because they could tell we were "Americans!" and maybe we had something, anything, to make their lives better in that moment. Then, on the coast, the most majestic beach I had ever seen, the white sand, warm, not hot, the clearest water. We had drinks on the beach. The vendors sold their authentic artifacts—handcrafted leather purses and shoes, metal art, crosses in stone. It's a part of the country we experienced but many homegrown Haitians may never see in their lifetime.

My father enjoyed the country and the adventure. He was intent on debunking the theory that as soon as you retire, you die. Having worked with children, youth, and families for thirty years, for the Commonwealth of Pennsylvania in the Department of Children and Youth, he could apply some of what he knew to the Haitians we were seeing.

While we were there, though, he started having pains. (I was too, but I ignored them in a way I knew I probably shouldn't; I was too focused on the mission.) Soon after we returned home, we discovered that Daddy had pancreatic cancer, one of the scariest kinds of cancer. But his grapefruit-sized tumor was removed by a renowned pancreatic surgeon, Dr. Charlie Yeo. Working with the transplant surgeon, Dr. Yeo took a vein from my father's kidney as part of the reconstruction, saving his life, thank God.

I soon found out the source of my own pain: I needed my gallbladder removed.

"You're beautiful on the outside but your insides are ugly," the surgeon commented matter-of-factly after the procedure.

I finally listened to my mentor, Dr. Ford: I kept my head down.

Sort of.

I did the work. I performed surgery as attending pediatric surgeon at Cooper, in Camden, New Jersey, while also running my concierge practice. I taught med students at Cooper. I was raising my three boys, of course, sharing custody with Matthew. Byron and I had become a couple. Though we weren't husband and wife, I appreciated how easily he accepted that my busy schedule was something I wasn't going to give up, because I felt it was my God-given responsibility to share what I could with people who would benefit from it. *Reach back to pull up.* My wings were outstretched.

The Cooper medical faculty hosted a fair on the importance of community screening. I was invited to speak at commencements, to appear on panels about women in science, to speak in praise of STEM (Science, Technology, Engineering, and Mathematics). My policy: If asked, I go. *Each one, teach one.* I devoted more attention to my nonprofit, It Takes Philly. I rejoiced when my Eagles won the Super Bowl.

Things were going fine. But the feeling that I could do more gnawed at me. Had I become too comfortable, living a suburban life? I was licensed as a surgeon in seven* states—Pennsylvania, New Jersey, New York, North Carolina, New Hampshire, Arizona, California—so I was all set, right? I knew I was an exception. My brother, Kamau, now an educator and a COO, was also an exception. The story of our lives is the story of exceptions. Was I doing all I should have been, all that God had put me here to do?

That's when I operated on Grace, the tiny little girl I wrote about at the beginning of this book. It was spring of 2018. I had operated before on newborns, many of them, though as a twenty-six-week-old preemie she may have been the youngest and smallest of all my patients. She was not the first child of color whose family came from the lowest socioeconomic rungs, and whose parent or parents reminded me

---

*I had let my license to practice in Delaware lapse since I did not anticipate working in the state.

of my own, or who made me imagine, as had Grace's mother, who I so easily could have become.

After Grace's operation, I kept in touch with her mom. As it is with every sick child I see, Grace had done nothing to deserve her situation. Her mother was almost certainly a victim of circumstance, too.

I operated again on Grace, an expected second surgery five months later. I was thrilled to see her doing well, very well.

But there was more I needed to do, for the other Graces of the world, and the other moms like Grace's mom. I could feel it.

My life at that time could go from newborns spectacularly surviving surgery to a movie star spectacularly jumping out of the sky.

Will Smith wanted me to be the medical professional on a special trip.

It's the job of a doctor to protect. Concierge medicine didn't change that.

In 2018, in March of his fiftieth birthday year, Will was getting his annual checkup when he learned of people bungee-jumping out of a helicopter. *I want to do that*, he thought. Approaching his milestone birthday, he planned to make his desire reality. His new life philosophy was to say yes to everything, which meant approaching things with no fear, including bungee-jumping out of helicopters—in this case, over the Grand Canyon. Networks were eager to broadcast it live. Will asked if I wanted to jump, too. I declined, mostly because I have three kids. Even if I didn't, though, I'm pretty sure I would have said no. I couldn't help asking his team, "Who are the pilots? Who's checking to make sure the pilots are healthy? Is there a copilot?" I wasn't the only adult in the room, but I had to do my job, annoying as I may have sounded. There were many things that I could not prevent from happening (you can use your imagination), but there are ways to lower the risk. I said that someone with flying knowledge should check on the pilots' experience. Make sure they weren't crazy. There would be a crew in the helicopter, and hopefully none of them would act stupidly. What if someone had a medical emergency while in flight? "Who's checking these people out?" I asked.

Will's production team hired me. I was up for the challenge.

Will asked me to take care of any and all potential medical needs. They had provided for an EMT, a good first step. But they were doing the exercise in Arizona, the desert. In some ways that would make for a better film shoot but in others made it more challenging. What kind of terrain would we be dealing with? Would snake bites be a problem? I researched possible dangers and put together a proposal for the production company about everything to prepare for. Retinal detachment can happen when you drop too fast and vision blurs; I considered having an ophthalmologist on-site to examine Will's eyes as soon as he landed. What about hypoxic episodes, from the oxygen-poor altitude? Were any of the women on the crew pregnant (yes), thus needing to avoid dehydration even more than the rest of us? Electricity would be scarce, as would bathrooms, gas, and running water. When I flew out there, I made sure everyone had medical clearance before they could participate as part of the flight crew—a physical exam plus a note from their personal physician that they were cleared for extreme sport activity. No high blood pressure, no increased risk of stroke while up there. I was also present for all the practice jumps in California before "The Jump" in Arizona.

It wasn't my job to tell Will not to jump out of a helicopter, only to keep him as safe as possible while he had the experience of a lifetime.

Afterward, he threw a big birthday party right there in the Grand Canyon, with amazing chefs and a great meal. There were tents and famous movie directors and everybody got T-shirts. Will knows how to have a good time.

As I looked around at the smiling faces, I couldn't help but smile myself. Will was happy and I was happy. Basically, I had put together a team in a very short amount of time and we'd built a triage hospital in the middle of the desert. Who does that?

I had no idea it was a dress rehearsal.

In the fall, Byron and I traveled to London to see our team, the Philadelphia Eagles, play an NFL game against the Jacksonville Jaguars at famed Wembley Stadium—the Eagles won!—and since we were already overseas, we decided to visit some other European cities. While we were enjoying an afternoon on a *bateau mouche*, one of those open boats that glide down the Seine as tourists admire the beauty of Paris around them, Byron got down on one knee. I had no idea what was happening. I was on my phone trying to get us tickets to the Louvre and he told me to get off the phone.

"But I'm doing something! I have to order them now!"

"Ala, put your phone down for once!"

When he took my hands in his, I started to realize something else was going on.

The roving singer began in on "La Vie en Rose." All the tourists seated nearby aimed their phones, then sent me the recording afterward. I have the marriage proposal on film from a half-dozen angles.

I still don't know how he got that over on me. Went to Europe to share time together and watch the Eagles, and came back engaged!

Sometime after the proposal, I was listening to WURD, the nation's oldest Black radio station, when they announced that Iyanla Vanzant would be appearing at the Quaker Meeting House off of South Street just before Christmas to celebrate twenty-five years since the publication of her amazing book, *Acts of Faith*.

It was a bright, festive day in Philadelphia, with snow on the ground. I attended the reading with my friend Leslie. There were hundreds of people in attendance. Ms. Vanzant delivered an inspirational speech that said, more or less: *We are not what happened to us.* She spoke about being on top of the world and also being at rock bottom. She spoke about her children.

Before she signed books, there was time for a few questions. My heart felt as if it was going to pound right out of my chest.

I stood in the pew, introduced myself to the author, and just dove in. "How do you forgive a person who was supposed to protect you? How do you coexist with a parent who you felt was involved in your being molested as a child? They learn about it and now they want to be your best friend, and life is just great and all . . . how do you move on? Everyone's moving like they were so instrumental in my success but they were also a big part of my pain. I'm still mad because you didn't protect me! Because you believed them over me! And you took their side and made me feel like it was my fault. You made yourself a priority over your child. But you were supposed to protect me."

I didn't bother to conclude with, *And that's why I chose such a difficult profession, where I put kids above all things, including myself.*

"What would you want that parent to say?" asked Ms. Vanzant.

I was slightly taken aback by her question.

"I don't know," I said, finally. "I guess I want them . . . to apologize? And say that they wish it didn't happen. She's told me, 'You're the best daughter ever, I'm proud of you.' Yet I can't get past the fact that during one of the most painful times in my life, I felt she chose herself over me. How do I come to grips with that?" It had taken me a long time to forgive and move on—it wasn't a straight line—and I realized I was not what happened to me. I was not to blame for what happened to me and would not allow myself to be defined by it. Did it still make me angry? Absolutely! But we all have to live with something.

"Okay, so I'm your mother," she said. "And I've just apologized for what happened. Do you feel better? Does that make it all go away?"

"No, not really," I said.

"It's not your mother that you need to address," she said. "It's younger Ala. She's the one. You have to tell her that none of this was her fault. The one to whom it happened. *You* have to tell *her* that it's okay. She did not ask for it. She did not want this to happen to her. That can't come from anyone but you." She paused. "Can you tell her that?" Maybe she saw skepticism in my eyes. "You have to forgive that child."

I was listening so hard to every word.

"And then let it go," said Ms. Vanzant. "Take a bath and just let it all go."

I cried and cried. Leslie cried. Close as we were, I had never told her about my past before that day. Many people from the audience came over to tell me they appreciated my comments. Only afterward did I stop to consider that I had opened up like that *publicly*, in front of hundreds of people listening in. Strangers.

The episode was therapeutic. It wasn't my fault. It wasn't young Ala's fault. Of *course* it wasn't. I needed to understand that—she needed to understand that—but for a long time I couldn't. I would go back and forth. I knew the "standard" process—striving to heal, remembering the abuse, knowing it wasn't my fault, then getting in touch with anger, then grief, then talking more about the abuse, then moving on and coming back. There were steps, but they didn't always go in one direction.

After opening up to Ms. Vanzant, I began to feel better. Just in that moment, it was done. I did not deserve what happened to me. Those who should have protected me failed me. At times that made me angry. But it didn't mean they didn't love me. Sometimes good people make bad decisions. I would not be defined by what others had done or failed to do. I would move on. I would be a living testimony that you can have joy and move beyond. I would and could trust myself and love myself and know that I was worthy of everything beautiful that came into my life.

Usually it's a question you get asked when you're a kid. But when someone at a social function asked me, "What do you want to be?"—a curious question, since I knew they knew I was a practicing pediatric surgeon—I was ready with the answer.

"Sanjay Gupta, 2.0," I said.

I revered Dr. Gupta as much as anyone in medicine. I had seen him on CNN. I admired how he traveled to Guinea and put himself in harm's way, even risking contracting the Ebola virus himself. Same with the Zika virus. Okay, so potentially contracting horrible diseases wasn't the part I wanted to emulate. But I respected what this surgeon was doing with his knowledge: thinking differently. Surgeons are trained to think innovatively because we so often deal with the unexpected; the problems we encounter are acute, requiring us at times to come up with an untried solution, fast. Sometimes you have to see what the mind doesn't even suspect. There are things you don't find in books, so you have to use all you know to come up with a new approach. Dr. Gupta communicated public health issues in novel ways that made people notice.

There was no shortage of public health crises that mattered deeply to me. Dr. Gupta's example inspired me to find those issues, and my voice. Did my response also have something to do with him being a person of color? Perhaps.

We surgeons are sometimes reduced to technicians—very high-level technicians but technicians all the same—and that doesn't have to be an insult. For a surgeon, to cut is to cure. One person at a time. Surgeons need to have a keen sense to identify the sick and the not sick, to prioritize, to triage, to treat. We must be masters of detail. We had better listen to all we're being told because that, too, can improve the course of disease without a scalpel. I am a healer. I have taken an oath to first do no harm; then to serve, to prevent disease, to promote health.

There were causes I was involved in, charities I donated to, racial inequities I was aware of, ones that everyone with open eyes is aware of. But I had no idea what was coming. No one did. No one. And that this shocking global catastrophe would unleash such a naked display of inequity and injustice—in 2020! Not 1950, not 1860, not 1770, but 2020!—with literal life-and-death consequences for a staggering number of people, old and young. It forced me and many of the people around me to look at things through even newer eyes.

Someone once told me, "Smooth seas don't make for strong sailors." Frankly, I would happily have given up some strength for more smoothness. Sign me up, right? But if the seas were going to be rough, then, damnit, we needed to be ready to handle them.

Everything was about to change. We would soon be living in a new world. The way to adjust to this change? With a plan. A new plan. And then use the lessons learned from that to start, finally, fulfilling a health care "promise" to all those people in this country for whom that word, for the longest time, seemed to have no meaning.

Part II

WHAT HEALING LOOKS LIKE

"The true soldier fights not because he hates what is in front
of him, but because he loves what is behind him."

—G. K. CHESTERTON

14

INVISIBLE MEN AND WOMEN

In 1985, a landmark government report on health care and race was published. Margaret Heckler, then secretary of health and human services in President Ronald Reagan's administration, commissioned a task force to produce the *Report of the Secretary's Task Force on Black and Minority Health*, which would come to be known as the Heckler Report. It was the first U.S. government documentation of health disparities among racial and ethnic minorities in our country. It was the first official acknowledgment that known health disparities were related specifically to the color of one's skin.

Among its findings, the report concluded that health disparities accounted for sixty thousand excess minority deaths per year compared to Caucasians, across the "Big Six": cancer; cardiovascular disease and stroke; substance misuse; diabetes; unintentional injuries (homicides and accidents); and infant mortality. The report led, a year later, to the establishment of the Office of Minority Health, at the U.S. Department of Health and Human Services.

That was a good thing.

But did it lead to an overhaul in how health care funding was apportioned? To a better, fairer way of providing equal access to resources for all citizens? To a true addressing of the social determinants of health, so that the cultural crime of health inequity could be solved at its root?

You make the call.

I was a teenager when the report came out close to forty years ago, and I wasn't paying attention. But most other people weren't paying attention either, then or since.

Should I be concerned?

That's what everyone wanted to know in the first weeks of 2020. For days my phone had been ringing with calls of panic about the coronavirus. For a while there in the U.S., it was harming only people who had traveled from China, so if you hadn't just come back from there or gotten very close with someone who had, you were presumed safe. And even if that *did* describe you, it seemed as if you were vulnerable only if you were in your eighties or older (not that that demographic should be dismissed).

Then the virus spread, along with media coverage of it, and the disease showed that it could also harm older folks on cruise ships. Then residents of nursing homes, specifically in and around Seattle, Washington. Then younger staff working at those nursing homes. Even there, though, it seemed as if you had to suffer from a laundry list of comorbid health conditions to be in real trouble.

Thursday, March 5, 2020, was the first day I addressed Covid-19 publicly, in a post on Instagram.

For my family and me, as for quite a few people—often richer, often whiter—things did not turn completely upside down when Covid-19 first appeared. Five days later I went on Instagram to explain the basics of the disease, dispel myths (including that African Americans were somehow resistant to the virus), and offer recommendations; that same day my twins celebrated their tenth birthday, at Olive Garden and GameStop. That day I also appeared as a guest on a radio show with WURD's Andrea Lawful-Sanders to discuss coronavirus. News reports were scary but still full of uncertainty—probably another way of saying we were in "hopeful disbelief." Panic helped no one. There were steps you could take.

Two days after that, March 12, the kids' school closed. Offices closed. All scheduled elective surgeries were canceled. I essentially shuttered my surgical practice, though I still teleconsulted with patients in my medical concierge business. Everyone in my neighborhood, as in most neighborhoods in America, was running out to stock up. Home Depot, Walmart. Gallons of water. Basically, grabbing whatever remained on the emptying shelves. Byron was a Costco shopper, so we already had a ton of toilet paper.

For the moment I had little to worry about. I didn't have to go into work. I provided medical advice and called in prescriptions over the phone. I had purchased the last freezer at our Home Depot, so we had two, stocked, and we had filled every cabinet, as well. We had a working washer and dryer. We had fast internet. We turned on the TV and, along with the children, settled into what we hoped would be a short hibernation. We were in the suburbs, a good ten miles from the heart of Philly. We had money in the bank. We had gas in the car. We had an au pair to help with the kids. We had a nice yard. Where I live, the streets are so wide you can walk them maskless and not come close to a neighbor breathing on you. The kids had their devices, happily chilling all day on their computers and phones, watching YouTube and Netflix. We spent lots of time in our pajamas. We did puzzles. To be honest, sheltering in place meant time spent as a family that I had always longed for. The kids were excited to be home. No one was pressed.

But I began to focus on images out of New York City, news stories accompanied by the terrifying sight of refrigerator trucks lined up, unmarked graves, mass burials near Rikers Island.

The calls to my cell phone were now constant. So many friends, and friends of friends, said they couldn't get tested. They were concerned that they had Covid-19 but were being turned away. Apparently, they weren't sick enough. Many of those who managed to get to a doctor found it almost impossible to follow the recommended protocols—work from home; shelter in place; stay away from the elderly and generally social distance—not because they were irresponsible but because their jobs, their financial situations, their multigenerational households, and other life circumstances prevented it.

In those last weeks of March, I was calling ERs several times a day on behalf of patients. "Hello, this is Dr. Ala Stanford. You've just turned away my patient, Mr. Wilson. I believe he has symptoms consistent with coronavirus disease and needs a test." My intervention enabled Mr. Wilson and others to get tested fast. The nurse or doctor on the other end said yes immediately. Many of them were empathetic. They promised to phone back once they had results, and did.

I didn't mind making the calls; I had time, since I was mostly stuck at home. All those people with symptoms deserved help—oxygen, pain relief medication, enforced bed rest, attention—plus some clarity, to know if they needed to isolate from family, to avoid crowds and mass transit, to stay home from work.

Every person for whom I called the ER ultimately tested positive. Every single one. No, they hadn't recently been in China or been around anybody who was, they were not nurses or health care workers or, for the most part, over sixty-five—most of the main high-risk groups that earned you a test in those early months. They were Black and they were coughing and they had fever and they were having trouble catching their breath and wasn't that enough to be moved into the high-risk category? The criteria for test eligibility were created for the white majority, not for the Black and brown minority.

The people who called me got seen. But there was a far, far bigger group of folks that did not have my number, or the number of any doctor they trusted. If the pandemic was this scary for me and my peers, what about the people who did *not* have regular access to a doctor?

The last day of March, I performed an emergency operation on a premature infant. By this time, I was more than a little fearful of being in the hospital because that's where doctors, nurses, and other health care workers kept getting infected, even as everyone took precautions. How could we not be anxious? Hospitals were the place where ambulances shuttled those severely sick with Covid-19. Surgeons always mask when performing surgery, but this time I wore an N95 plus a 3-ply mask over that, with eyeglasses and a face shield. You shouldn't worry about yourself, only the patient, but at that extraordinary time the rules had changed. It's damn hard to practice social distancing when you're saving someone's life. My team and I were gathered in the typical close confines of an operating room created in the NICU— nurses and residents, neonatologist, respiratory therapist. We were all at risk from each other. We needed to protect the newborn from further harm. She had a perforated intestine. The surgery lasted just over an hour. It went well.

It was one of the last operations I would perform for the next three years. There were things to address more important even than that.

To a surgeon, to cut is to cure. To a doctor, a patient advocate, a community activist, a social justice warrior, a leader—pick your preferred title—you cure by identifying the problem, devising a solution, finding your tribe (those who believe in your vision), refusing to take "no" for an answer, and never losing sight of your goal: to save lives.

In those last dark days and nights of March 2020 and the very first ones of April, I watched Anderson Cooper on CNN religiously at 8 p.m. As more and more images flashed by of people who had died of Covid-19, I noticed that so many of them were public-facing employees, and so many of them were Black. I figured that what was true nationally was true locally. There were no demographic data yet from my city or state, so the observations I was making were not yet substantiated by hard facts.

On April 3, I opened *The Philadelphia Tribune*, a Black-owned newspaper, and looked in horror at the data. Black people in Philadelphia *were* catching Covid-19 and dying at rates far out of proportion to their numbers. Steven Brown, a research associate at the Urban Institute, captured the reality: "When white America catches a cold, Black America catches pneumonia." My old community, filled with people who looked like me, from the streets where I grew up, was suffering on a whole other level. People could not get medical care until they were so sick that their trips to hospital emergency rooms were one-way, followed by a final journey to the morgue.

"Coronavirus was like a heat-seeking missile" for Black people, journalist Yamiche Alcindor, host of PBS's *Washington Week*, said later. Dr. Neel T. Shah, assistant professor of obstetrics, gynecology and reproductive biology at Harvard Medical School, put it this way: "Covid-19 divided the world into people who could protect themselves and those who could not."[1] Those who could not were much more likely to be persons of color.

Why? Isn't a virus agnostic? An equal-opportunity infector and killer?

Well, no,

- not if the social determinants of health—access to healthy food, a decent education, reliable quality health care, money, a safe neighborhood, many of the prime forces that largely shape whether people live in good health—are not equal;
- not if unofficial but very real policies like redlining have kept the social determinants of health unequal for generations;
- and not if political leaders continue to make decisions based on the best interests of some, or even the few, rather than everyone, particularly those most in need.

A few days after I read that story in the *Tribune*, Dr. Anthony Fauci, the most public member of the White House Coronavirus Task Force, the longtime director of the National Institute of Allergy and Infectious Diseases and later the chief medical advisor to the president, delivered a Covid-19 briefing at the White House. After he finished speaking, he returned to the podium to respond to a question about the effect of the virus on the African American community. He wanted to make two points about why Blacks were more harmed than whites by the virus:

1. Racial inequities in the American health care system had always been there and were still there; and
2. Blacks suffered a higher rate of comorbidities, particularly those that made Covid-19 more lethal—diabetes, obesity, hypertension, asthma.

That was my "aha" moment.

I was grateful to have a voice of science and reason acknowledge that the health disparities were rooted in systemic racism. People needed to hear that. (Though I was not so naïve to think that everyone who heard it would accept it.) But Dr. Fauci's second statement troubled me. In fact, I felt a vague sense of PTSD, an echo from my first year of medical school, back when I listened as case studies were recounted and the reason for the patient's poor health—often the Black patient's poor health—was ascribed, at least in part, to his or her lack of personal responsibility. Back when I was a young medical student, I felt helpless to raise any objections to the way "those people" were being portrayed, though it was misleading and perpetuated bias. Now, a quarter-century later, at the dawn of a global health pandemic, as a doctor with years of experience, I was less comfortable remaining quiet. What Dr. Fauci said was true but unintentionally damning. Yes, Blacks suffered from diabetes, obesity, hypertension, and asthma at a higher rate than whites did; I knew the numbers only too well. I deeply respect Dr. Fauci the scientist. And while I was glad he called out our health care system for its racism, he should have noted that *the increased rate of comorbidities in Blacks was a consequence of systemic and institutionalized inequity.* Without connecting those dots, too many were free to think: *Well, they wouldn't be suffering as much if they'd only taken better care of themselves.*

There was no way we were going to fix what was fundamentally wrong with the system if a significant number of people believed that personal responsibility, or the lack of it, was at the heart of the problem.

I felt a surge of anger. As a Black doctor I felt empowered finally to challenge this depiction of my own. I was in tears talking on the phone to Kamau. "We have to do something," I told him.

I went from being comfortably sheltered at home to deeply uncomfortable.

People were calling me with more stories of frustration. (I know that so many people, of all races and classes, felt confused, scared, and frustrated in those early months of the pandemic.) These were some of the reasons Black Philadelphians were being turned away by hospitals for tests, aside from their not being in a high-risk group:

You don't have a referral from a doctor.

You don't have a scheduled appointment.

We're just so inundated.

The more I spoke with those in authority, the more I heard complaints and "explanations" that the people dying at such astonishing rates were actually dying thanks to their comorbid conditions, like high blood pressure and diabetes.

"But couldn't it also be that by the time they get access to the ER," I asked those who should know, on several occasions, "they've got one foot in the grave because they're so damn sick?"

"Maybe," came one answer, flatly.

Enraging. It was a funhouse of mirrors except there was nothing fun about it.

On April 7, I read this headline: "Positive Tests Higher in Poorer Neighborhoods Despite Six Times More Testing in Higher-Income Neighborhoods."

So many people languished in sickness for days before they got help. Through social media, radio appearances, and on phone calls I offered the advice that most informed doctors did: Hydrate to keep your fever under control. Yes to acetaminophen, no to ibuprofen. If you can get your hands on a pulse oximeter to measure your oxygen saturation, do. It was mostly a respiratory illness, so dropping O_2 levels indicated more serious sickness. If you can't find a pulse oximeter because everyone is grabbing those up, here's a test: If you need a couple extra breaths to get through a sentence, or you're out of breath walking to the kitchen, get to a hospital. If you can't do that, then lie on your stomach in the prone position. If you have a bacterial pneumonia on top of the virus—assuming you can get in to see someone who could actually check for that—then you need antibiotics. As we all learned very quickly, there were no antivirals, no magic pill. That's what made Covid-19 so scary and deadly.

Then there was the communal problem: So many of the sick or possibly sick were bus drivers, police officers, sanitation workers, nurses and home health aides, grocery store clerks—people who worked among the public, who couldn't just decide to take off work without cause. Or do their jobs from home. Or shelter in place. Through no fault of theirs, they were spreading Covid-19 at lightning speed. And these jobs were being done by people of color at a higher rate than by white people.

Outside of hospitals, there were no testing sites in the 'hood. Philly is a commuter city. Technically, the Black people I was reading about could go to the suburbs. Take the train, a couple trains, maybe a couple buses out to where physicians were, maybe somewhere on the Main Line ... but there, too, they were often turned away. Their doctor wasn't on staff. No script. (Why? Because they had no doc, period. Why? Because of repeated disappointment, mistreatment, and being ignored by the very same health care system.) Not over sixty-five. Doesn't look that sick. Not a health care worker. Not in a car.

Yeah, please let that last one sink in. *There's* a real solid reason for worsening a public health crisis: Refuse to test people who are likely infected and suffering and spreading it and who are also doing their civic duty by taking a half-day off from work and losing hours of pay to take public transportation to a distant testing site . . . yeah, *don't* test those people because they're not in their own vehicle.

It got overwhelming. I was on the phone with hospitals all day every day. I was hearing of families where the kids had been orphaned. Will Smith reached out to me. "Ala, I need a pandemic plan." He wanted to know how best to protect his family, what to stock up on, what to avoid in the event someone got infected, where was the safest place to be. Other concierge patients also wanted to know. They had options. I had options. We could all practice social distancing and keep our core group small, stay in our bubble, avoid crowds until we absolutely couldn't. We rarely couldn't.

The people dying mostly lived in a density I knew well from when I was a little girl. Now those neighborhoods were Petri dishes of lethal disease. I had punched my way out of there and now had a blessed career and a large backyard with grass and trees. I was even starting to build up what some might call generational wealth. I had moved on.

But then I hadn't. I couldn't. Once again, America was failing Black people.

15

BLACK DOCTORS

In 2020, Black people comprised 44 percent of the population of Philadelphia but 52 percent of Covid deaths. African Americans were (and are) the largest racial group in the city. Of the twenty-five largest cities in America, Philadelphia was (and is) the poorest.[1] Many of its Black citizens are working-class. They were at the back of the bus.

It angers me that triage thinking, or some humane version of it, was not in play in the early terrifying days of the pandemic. Ideally, the group that's hurting the most should be a target for resource allocation. This isn't just my idealistic view of the world; it's how you respond in a public health emergency. The people who were suffering most were not first on the list. I don't know where on the list they were, but it didn't seem like second or third either. I understood that there were constraints on testing, that frail elderly people and those living and working in nursing homes were considered the most vulnerable groups. I got it. Those people needed and deserved our attention. But whatever resources were left over did *not* go to the large, vulnerable Black population that was suffering and dying in such shocking numbers—in Philly and elsewhere. The results of a study published later that spring

showed that counties in the U.S. with Black populations higher than
the national average (13.4 percent) had death rates as much as three
times higher than for counties with Black populations lower than the
national average.[2]

And it was not just about being poor. The multiplier in that study
remained largely the same regardless of income or the rate of comorbid conditions. It proved a point that so many of us had been trying
to make for a long time: Disparities are not just the result of socioeco-
nomics. *Poor people, poor outcomes*: Yes, that's undoubtedly true for poor
Black and poor brown and poor white folks. But many studies have
shown that bad health outcomes have at least as much to do with the
color of your skin as your income or health insurance plan.

If only my city's Public Health Department had followed its own
stated goal, the city and the fate of so many of its residents, particularly its Black ones, would have been different: "The mission of the
Department of Public Health is to protect and promote the health of
all Philadelphians and to provide a safety net for people who are disproportionately impacted by societal factors that limit their access to
health care and other resources necessary for optimal health." As the
public health crisis grew, that phrase, "disproportionately impacted,"
should have applied to more Black people, poor and not.

I could not live in anger. It helped no one. I had to turn all this into
action.

Early in April I talked with Jada Pinkett Smith, who mentioned
that the actor Sean Penn had funded a mobile unit in California to test
people for Covid.[3]

I wondered how feasible that would be in Philly, particularly in
colder temperatures.

But then I thought . . . That might work! Going to the people! A
mobile unit that could be brought into the community!

I formulated a plan. I needed to create an organization whose purpose was clear: a group of medical professionals going around testing

Philadelphians that were most impacted by Covid. I wouldn't assume that because I was a Black doctor, Black Philadelphians would automatically trust me. My group would have to earn the people's trust.

Black Doctors COVID-19 Consortium.

That was the name that came to me. Why not? It was about time, I thought, that a health care initiative answered a need that had for far too long been ignored. Black people were so often an afterthought in the American health care system. In the midst of Covid, Black people were the ones disproportionately affected, and the name I came up with connoted acknowledgment. It said, *We see you. We hear you.* Not to diminish the harrowing effect of Covid-19 on Asian people or Latino people or other brown people or working-class white people or any white people . . . but this was about Black people. The numbers in the community were staggering. To make the organization name so intentional was to address what so many Black people feel: that the traditional medical establishment is untrustworthy. Black patients had better outcomes when treated by Black doctors rather than white doctors.[4] It's just a fact, a sad fact. Incredibly, new data showed, as I wrote earlier, that having even one Black doctor on a hospital staff improves health outcomes for Black patients.[5] Can you believe that? So if anyone thought the inclusion of "Black" in the name was too radical or exclusive or racist? Look around. The name was clear, honest, and practical. For Black people, I wanted it to connote trustworthiness. I wanted the Black community to know that we as licensed Black doctors and Black health care professionals were coming to help (though I assumed I'd recruit non-Black staff, too). For everyone else, I wanted the name to convey that we existed out of necessity. Because the institutions designed to provide and protect Black people from this disease were failing.

I also liked the name because I created it. I sought no one's permission. I was tired of seeking approval from people. I was tired of getting thwarted.

I checked online to make sure the URL was available. (Of course it was.) I also purchased the domain blackdoctorsconsortium.com, because there would come a time when this entity was no longer primarily about Covid-19.

Because I had started my nonprofit, It Takes Philly, years earlier, I already had the 501(c)(3) designation and documentation. I made BDCC a subsidiary of It Takes Philly, Inc., to simplify and quickly provide infrastructure.

Black Doctors would have a mobile testing unit—unless we didn't have to. True, so far the Philadelphia city and Pennsylvania state governments had underwhelmed me and everyone else who looked like me. Where were the Covid testing sites in Black neighborhoods? But maybe—*maybe*—with some prodding, they would rise to the occasion. And Black Doctors COVID-19 Consortium would need to provide only secondary support.

And ... no.

I reached out to every city and state official I could think of—the health commissioner, the mayor, state senators, congresspeople and local officials, requesting information about how they were addressing the crisis among Black Philadelphians. I called, I emailed, I sent letters. *What's the plan? What are the resources? What's being done? How can I help? Do you know how many people are dying?* I don't know if the last of these questions, urgent as it was, particularly endeared me to the recipient.

All the answers I got back amounted to *Thanks, no thanks* and *Sorry* and *Not much*. I heard some version of: *Yeah, it does suck. Yeah, it is a shame.* Lots of empathy, and lots of arms up in the air, helpless. But also clueless. *Yes, Dr. Stanford, we agree wholeheartedly with you that it's unfortunate that this is happening.* One big shrug emoji.

The clock was ticking so I switched strategies. I didn't ask them what they were doing but told them what *I* was planning to do and maybe they could help?

On April 10, I discussed with a Pennsylvania state senator the problems, my intentions, and what I needed. I hoped my irritating persistence would light a fire and they would do what I, a private citizen who happened to be a licensed doctor, should not have had to. The day after, I followed up by email.

April 11, 2020

Dear Senator:

Below is a summary of each topic we discussed 4-10-20 aimed at reducing morbidity and mortality associated with coronavirus in African Americans.

- *Neighborhood Testing Station: Satellite COVID19 testing in African American communities hardest hit from COVID19. People are unable to have testing performed and be screened or are being turned away from testing sites and emergency departments. ASK: (1) To work in conjunction with city health workers, (2) testing supplies and media reagent, testing slips and protocol for lab drop off and results acquisition, (3) volunteers assist in operating the satellite unit. Tents for inclement weather. Vehicles for pop-up testing, i.e., back of passenger van; The goal of how many tests performed per week will depend on the amount of personnel, PPE and testing supplies. (Commissioner Farley and Health Department)*
- *Patients after being referred to hospitals or testing centers, with an order or prescription from a doctor and have been turned away upon arrival. They have also been turned away at drive-by testing as they did not have a car. ASK: Black Doctors COVID-19 Consortium physicians request "access" to refer patients to testing centers in each region in the city*

after deeming that a patient needs to be tested or admitted without
in-network/out-of-network restrictions, especially since no cost
is incurred to the hospital for the test. (Hospital Association and
Mayor's Office)

• Many African Americans live in multigenerational households. If a
person becomes COVID19 positive it is challenging to separate that
individual from other members of the household and therefore the
disease can spread to all members of the family from young to old
persons.
ASK: Housing in hotels and dormitory dwellings in Philadelphia
and Montgomery County for those with COVID19 for a
minimum of 14 days after diagnosis and symptoms have cleared.
(Commissioner Farley and Health Department)

• Supplies and personal protective equipment: PPE for drive-through
workers and food handlers, grocery store and pharmacy clerks,
Walmart and Target (e.g., type stores), sanitation, postal workers,
and SEPTA drivers. All entities where workers are in constant

You get the idea. My messages might as well have just faded away.
There was no immediate response. Nothing was happening, but I was
mastering the art of the follow-up letter. I wanted to create a chain
of correspondence—my questions and offers of help, their follow-up
rebuffing or silence.

One state senator responded that he couldn't do much. He lacked
the power to move things quickly because of the bureaucracy. I was
chasing my own tail. Once it was obvious that the people in supposed
authority were not responding fast enough, especially given the rapid-
ity of the spread and lethality of the disease, I switched gears: I would
call the hospitals and Federally Qualified Health Centers (FQHCs)
since they were the ones testing people.

I asked them if they were really turning people away and, if so, why?
They were not patients in our hospital system.
They did not have insurance.

They did not have an order or a script.

They were too young.

They did not have chronic health conditions.

They were not health care workers.

They were not in cars and we don't take walk-ups for testing.

I yelled, "But so many of them are symptomatic! They're probably positive!"

That's when I realized: *I guess we're doing this.*

I never checked to see how much money I had in my bank account; I just went online and started pricing van rentals. Through my own medical practice, I had access to PPE (personal protective equipment)—gowns, gloves, masks. I went to my office and scooped up all the equipment I could find. I had some extra supplies left over from the last mission trip to Haiti. I reached out to other physicians who had PPE, though their stashes weren't as plentiful as I'd hoped; hospitals were rightfully commandeering most of the supply, and for many doctors there was a "survival of the fittest" attitude. Hoarding was common. I was grateful for the support of some of my neighbors who were doctors—surgeons, anesthesiologists, fertility specialists. Like me, none of them were operating because surgery centers were closed. It was not uncommon to come home and find PPE on my doorstep. No note, just supplies, a response to an earlier text message.

Next, I needed test kits and a lesson on how to administer them. I called a physician friend who had performed tests. She walked me through the process, explaining how the specimens were kept on ice and how often she and her staff "decontaminated" for their own safety and that of the test-takers. Another friend, a family practice doctor who had closed down his office for the pandemic, offered me test kits. His nurse left all his extras in a box outside his office for me to pick up.

As a doctor with my own practice, in network with insurance companies as well as the companies that supplied the tests, I hoped to get more—lots more. I called LabCorp, one of the test providers. They didn't quite get what I was doing. "You're a surgeon, not a primary care physician," the person said. "We can't allocate them to you. They'll expire."

"No, no! I'll use them! If you send them to me, I will use them. Please give me a chance."

They said no.

I called again, explaining the situation with more detail and passion. They said no.

At the time, they wanted $50 a test (later it would go up to $100). It didn't sit right with me that a person might not know that he or she was positive and endanger others in their circle because they couldn't afford a $50 test. I would cover it, but I hoped insurance would cover me.

I called the lab again. This time the representative asked me who was going to pay for the tests. My response: "Bill me directly, please." Finally, they relented, and sent five hundred tests.

Next, I needed medical professionals. I recruited a couple of doctors I respected greatly—Dr. Pierre Chanoine and Dr. Renell Dupree. Both were available; both had offices that had temporarily closed. I messaged Dr. Velma Scantlebury (a surgeon and a mentor from Pitt), who worked with the Student National Medical Association, telling her I needed medical school volunteers for mobile unit testing going door-to-door in Philadelphia. Covid-19 was keeping so many med students home from their rotations, just months before graduation. I thought back to the excitement of those weeks right before my own graduation from medical school and wondered, *How frustrating must it be for them now?* There were young first-, second-, and third-year doctors, too, sitting at home watching the public health crisis unfold, eager to help.

Dr. Scantlebury and SNMA helped me recruit a couple medical students from the Philadelphia College of Osteopathic Medicine (PCOM)—Natalie Gonzalez, a fourth-year, and Dana Heller, a third-year.

I recruited Byron.

Meanwhile, I had my mom rent a white van for transportation and supply storage. I instructed her to please *not* tell the rental company what we planned for the van; in that atmosphere, April 2020, who knew if they would have declined to rent it to us? It cost about three grand a month. It wouldn't be long before my credit cards were maxed out. Byron's, too.

I got the word out on my professional websites and my social media: If you want to get tested, email me with your information, and we, Black Doctors COVID-19 Consortium, will come to you!

We had an organizational name, proper registration, a van, tests, PPE, and a professional and committed staff. We had a list of people who wanted us to come test them. We had a zoom call on Wednesday, April 15, 2020. The next day, we headed into the city.

16

THE CHURCH PARKING LOT IS MY NEW OR

A frigid Thursday, miserable and gray and spitting icy rain. We were three doctors—a pediatrician, a family physician, and me—plus two medical students. The students were not licensed to test but could register patient information and help in other important ways. Byron was our driver. Altogether that made six of us in the white van.

We convened at our home church, Salem Baptist, in Abington, Montgomery County.

In the sanctuary, I talked the team through the plan. We had ice and coolers for the specimens, and PPE to keep ourselves safe. I showed the team the test kits. Dr. Dupree showed us how to package the specimens. The med students would be in charge of packaging and labeling. We reviewed the list of patients whose homes we would be visiting. Pastor Marshall Mitchell quickly devised the most efficient route, starting with those located furthest away, in South and West Philly, and working our way back to our home base of Salem Baptist.

We discussed how to decontaminate when we were finished for the day. We looked at each other. Then it seemed appropriate, natural, for us to lock arms, bow our heads and pray, led by Reverend Mitchell. We were parked at a church, our church, and we needed protection, mercy, and grace. In that gray and rainy moment, it hit me that we were going toward what many were running from.

Reverend Mitchell, in his car, led the way to the first patient since he had created the route. I was grateful for his presence. It felt a little like when we were doing medical mission work in Haiti. He also had the forethought to inform the media about what we were doing and to begin taking pictures and video.

Five hours later, I couldn't exactly call our first day a success. It was more like a day of learning.

We drove all over Philly. Each person on our list came out of their home. We tested them right there on the sidewalk, got back in the van, and drove to the next location. My idea of going *to* the people turned out to be absurdly time-consuming. Our fierce, professional, committed team tested a whopping total of twelve people that day.

12.

At the end of the day, back at Salem Baptist, we debriefed. Twelve people a day wasn't going to cut it. My idea of going house-to-house was not exactly optimal.

"That was good," I said, trying to spin it positively, "and exhausting." After a pause, I admitted, "Okay, this is not going to work."

We needed a reset. I had to take a step back and remember my own young life. Where did my community naturally gather?

The churches.

The Black church is the one institution that we own and control. It has long been a place of hope, caring, and love. If we were going to impact people, it needed to be on their terms—our terms—and the Black church has always been that place. It had an integrity. And many of these church buildings are old, more than a century. These were not fly-by-night structures, and ours was not going to be a fly-by-night operation. People in the Black community tend to trust and respect their pastors and their churches, even those who are not members. They know that the church is a safe place.

Aside from trustworthiness and centrality, churches offered other advantages: parking lot, electricity, and restrooms.

I got immediate and essential support, as always, from Reverend Mitchell. He was well-known and highly regarded in the community, minister of the largest church outside of the city. His grandfather, biracial and Jewish, had come to the Philadelphia area from Virginia at the turn of the twentieth century, married a Black woman, then pastored Black Baptist churches in the region. His own father had pastored until he was eighty-nine. Pastor Mitchell would help with the bureaucratic parts of our operation. He had the relationships, and he knew city politics. The medical stuff was my department.

On Friday we strategized on next steps. We needed to go where the Covid positivity rate was highest. Drawing on my research experience, I scoured the Philadelphia Department of Public Health website for testing positivity numbers; it was not easily found so I created a table myself, highest to lowest. The top five:

ZIP CODE	% POSITIVE TEST	% AFRICAN AMERICAN
19126	44.4	83.4
19141	40.8	84.4
19151	37.1	87.9
19139	36.4	88.6
19150	35.2	94.1

I asked Pastor Mitchell to find a church in each zip code. Or several. That became our roadmap. We would go to where the need was greatest. We would follow the data. In academia, we call it "evidence-based practice."

As promised, Reverend Mitchell called pastors of churches in the zips with the highest Covid-positive rates.

"Miller Memorial says we can come tomorrow," he said after he finished another call. I posted the details of our planned appearance on Instagram, Facebook, and my concierge practice website. BDCC didn't have a website yet; to be fair, we were all of two days old!

We could do better than twelve people a day. We had to.

APRIL 18

Saturday. Another cold, overcast day, this time at Miller Memorial Baptist Church in North Philly—Pastor Damaris Walker's church. This time, no more door-to-door.

I'd spent the preceding thirty-six hours recruiting: I had sent texts to health care professionals and got on Zooms with doctors and medical students, welcoming one and all to join us. I found out who was available, who was comfortable doing testing, who wasn't—and oh, yeah, please bring PPE if you have it! When our van pulled up to the church at seven that Saturday morning, nearly every one of the doctors and surgeons I'd contacted was there. Twenty licensed physicians and ten med students. So many familiar faces standing outside in the cold gray morning. Sure, they had spare time now that their private practice offices were shut down, but still . . . I got choked up seeing how many people wanted to help. Everyone had brought PPE.

We were all bundled up. Testing inside the church would have been a lot toastier, but far riskier. We couldn't chance a superspreader event. And our first church setting had to go well for other churches to open their doors, their parking lots, their side streets to us. We set up outside.

This time we tested 150 people. Way better than twelve people. But even so, we would have to get far more efficient to have a fighting chance against this virus.

APRIL 20

We tested at Enon Tabernacle Baptist, Pastor Alyn Waller's church, the largest predominantly Black congregation and one of the most respected churches in the city.

We were slated to start at eight in the morning. By 7:30, more than a hundred cars were lined up. *If you build it*, as they say, *they will come*. The sight confirmed for me that we were exactly where we needed to be.

Many of the cars were loaded with four, five, six people. Full vans. Families, adults with their elderly parents. Of those in packed vehicles, I wondered: *Did they all have Covid already or were they spreading it to everyone in the car?* In addition to drive-up service, we also offered walk-up for those who came by foot or bus. We had chairs along the sidewalk. We had four hundred tests so when the line reached that many people, we closed it. No point making people wait in line for hours when we knew we didn't have enough tests.

So many of the people we saw were anxious, many outright scared. Many didn't realize how communicable Covid was. They didn't know if they were sick with it, or with just a regular cold, or infected but asymptomatic. Or not infected at all. They wanted to protect their parents and their children. Everyone wanted to tell us what had brought them there.

"I just buried my brother with Covid and we're back from the graveside. Maybe I have it too."

"My husband has a breathing tube in the hospital. We can't visit, it's hard to get information, but we wonder if the rest of the family has it."

"My mom, husband, and kids have it and I think I gave it to them."

The whole transaction, from the time a car pulled up to the testing area to the time we sent patients on their way, took ten to fifteen minutes, depending on the number of people in the car. When each test was done, we instructed the patient to go home and quarantine until their results came back. In many cases, that didn't go over well.

"You kidding? I gotta go to work."

"I just came to get my test on my *way* to work."

"Can't stay home. Too many mouths to feed."

We tested everyone. Children, seniors, all those in between. A man posted on Instagram a video of himself getting tested, and more cars showed up, the line growing longer and longer. A news van arrived from Channel 6, the ABC affiliate.

For many of the people we saw that day, guidance from the CDC and the White House was not helpful. The Black men and women from these zip codes in Philadelphia worked in the post office, in grocery stores, for SEPTA, driving the bus, operating the train. They were electricians and plumbers. Even if one couldn't care less about Black people, their contributions were essential. If they didn't continue showing up at work and decided instead to stay home and take care of themselves or quarantine just in case, Philadelphia would grind to a halt. They were keeping their city going, our nation, like so many other times in American history. The sacrificial lambs. America wouldn't be able to go anywhere, go shopping, get food delivered, get lots of services we wanted or needed. These essential people were now rolling down their car windows so that my team and I, in our quasi-hazmat suits and with our nasal swabs, could test them for a wildly virulent disease.

That day our team used every last one of our four hundred tests. As we were finishing up, the LabCorp people came by to pick up the specimens. We watched the exchange carefully, ensuring chain of custody.

When the results were in (two to three days later), approximately one hundred of the four hundred people we tested at Enon Tabernacle that day were positive, 25 percent. One of the positives was Enon's own Pastor Waller. He went on Facebook Live and shared the news with everyone. He hadn't planned to test, but did so to set an example for his congregation. And damn if he wasn't positive. Many in the congregation were devastated to learn he had it. Many were freaked out because they had attended his indoor service the Sunday prior.

To this day, when we speak about the early days of Covid-19, Pastor

Waller will tell me, "Remember that time you came to my church and gave me Covid?" I always give him a hug and a side-eye.

APRIL 22

Pinn Memorial Baptist Church, in West Philadelphia, and formerly Pastor Mitchell's father's church. Here we tested police officers on their beat. They pulled up and we tested them in their cop cars, because they were on their shifts. Days later, when we got back the results and one of them—Black, mid-thirties—was positive, I called to tell him. He was beside himself—not because he had Covid, but because he had gotten a test without first clearing it with his commanding officer. "Well, you need to take off from work for at least a few days, for your benefit and those of the people you work with," I said. "Think of your partner, the people you're protecting and serving. If you want, have your CO call me and I'll tell them myself." The officer was not the only person, by far, who got tested with some hesitation: Many folks felt it was better not knowing they were positive, especially if they were asymptomatic, since there was no one to fill their spot. Lots of people worked jobs that provided no sick pay, so no work meant no income. And lots of people who *did* get sick pay didn't feel right taking time off while their colleagues were in the thick of it.

APRIL 24

The line of cars leading to the Mount Airy Church of God in Christ parking lot wrapped around one block, then another, what seemed like for miles. When we arrived, the lot was filled with cars.

Oh, my God, I thought. We hadn't even parked the van or figured out the best way to manage the day and the site. Word must have spread, particularly after Pastor Waller's Facebook post, and now things had exploded. It showed not only how much we were needed but also that we were building trust, a true blessing. And we gave that love right back to them. We always showed compassion to the people we tested—it was a privilege to be their health care provider—and often we were asked to pray with some of the older folks, before the test. I couldn't help but think of how grateful I had always felt for the blessing and privilege of being a pediatric surgeon. For all that I did to help the children, they did more to help me. I felt that again now, with each test I performed, to get thanks from all these people, young and especially old, acting as if *I* were the one performing all the good and deserving of thanks. My mentor Dr. Ford used to say, "The days of 'thank you's,' 'good job's,' and pats on the back will soon be over. You'll have to be your own judge of a job well done." In surgery, you can tell a good operation by the improvement in a patient's health. Here, I could tell we were doing well by the volume of people showing up each day and, eventually, what I hoped would be a steady decrease in the positivity rate. The community itself promoted us and validated what we were doing.

Natalie Gonzalez, one of our brightest volunteers, organized the paperwork and administrative tasks. She wasn't a doctor yet so she couldn't do testing, but she set up tables, designated teams, came up with a system. "The only thing the doctor should be doing is administering the test and handing the specimen to you," I instructed Natalie. She helped with registration, which was painstaking and so important. She was a keeper.*

The whole staff was inspiring. So many talented, committed young people, quick learners, who then imparted their knowledge to other young people. This was a community story as much as a public health crisis story. I had known one of our nurses, Shelah, for years because I'd operated on her daughter when she was three months old. Now, more than a decade later, Shelah had heard my name on a segment for a local radio station, called the phone number she had for me from years before, and asked how she could help. And here she was, helping.

---

*Her medical school graduation, held virtually, fell on a testing day, so we created a makeshift ceremony for her—theme music, I hooded her, she flung her hat in the air, a special moment for us all. Natalie would work with BDCC through July, when she started her internship in pediatrics. She is now a fellow in neonatology.

The team collected insurance information on a demographic intake form because LabCorp had advised me to. I was hesitant at first to ask for such info: I didn't want anyone to feel shame for having to write down that they had no insurance. Nor did I want to erode trust by making them wonder, *If this is free testing, why do they need my insurance info?* It was just in case at a later time I could be reimbursed.

(I was fortunate to be a LabCorp client in good standing. They sent the testing kits, and soon after processing I received invoices for payment of thousands and thousands of dollars. At the time I was not sure where I would get the money to pay them, but I was not focused on that while we were saving lives.)

For undocumented citizens or those with housing insecurity, we needed a name and phone number or some other way to contact them with their test results; if they had no reliable contact info, we gave them *our* number and future location schedule so they could find us for results.

We tested Black people and anyone who was in line regardless of race or ethnicity. The lone requirement was that you had been exposed to Covid-19 and were thus at risk of infection.

As on previous days, almost each person we tested at Mount Airy was appreciative. "It feels so good to have someone who looks like me helping me," said one middle-aged Black woman, "and who's a doctor."

We had a few nurses in line who said they couldn't get tested at work. (Yep, you read that right.) I heard too many stories of people employed in health care (e.g., at dialysis units) who said they were *sure* they had Covid—that everyone they worked with probably had it— but so what? What difference did it make? Their presence at work was essential. Being at work could save a life—yet jeopardize their own. More than one nurse told me that their supervisor instructed them not to test. "If you're out with Covid," said one supervisor, "who will get these patients on hemodialysis?"

For them, it was: Why test if it doesn't change anything? If, positive or negative, you still have to go to work? Unless you were so sick you couldn't get up? There was no in-between. *If you're not in the hospital, you'd better be IN the hospital.*

Many people at the church that day appeared very sick—and not just the elderly. Some were so sick, by the time we called to give them their positive results, they were in the hospital or deceased.

Quite a few people on line had just returned from cemeteries. Many cried. "I have a friend in the hospital and my mom just died from Covid . . ." They had trouble going on. How could they, when they were prevented from talking or seeing or touching or advocating for their loved ones in what would be those last terrible days and hours? When their parents or grandparents or spouses or partners or siblings were quarantined in hospitals, many of them never to make it out? How terrifying to imagine. My team and I had to be strong for the people we were serving. We were there not just to test and explain but to listen. I knew, as a surgeon—as a human being—that lots of times patients need a listening ear. Not just your skill and the scalpel and the medication but your heart and soul and understanding. So many of the people in line weren't medically savvy and didn't know what to believe; in those early days of the pandemic, few did, including experts. Reassurance and genuine eye contact counted for a lot. Our team was good at remaining calm and educating people. Information, accurate information, reduced the fear. So did our transparency. All of it was encircled by faith. *You're not alone. You matter.* That emotionally present approach helped to dissipate a lot of anxiety. For many, we were the first touch they were able to have with any health care person.

Late in the day a woman approached me. She introduced herself as the pastor of another church in the city and handed me a check made out to Black Doctors COVID-19 Consortium for five hundred dollars. "What you're doing is so important," she said.

She looked like she could really use the money herself. She was the first person who gave to BDCC.

For some of the staff volunteers, the whole testing experience was less inspiration than rude awakening. It was impossible not to note the sheer inequality of health care attention that Black people routinely get. One young Black woman, a city emergency worker who lived minutes from Mount Airy, told me after the day was done, "I knew there was implicit bias against the underserved community, which is why I volunteered, but I didn't know how profound until the pandemic came along." Seeing those hundreds of cars, people waiting in line for hours, the racial makeup, brought it home. It angered her and many others. Me too. "It really is about race," she said. "There's no other reason." Her awakening was typical—depressing in the moment, maybe, but perhaps constructive in the long run.

As on previous days, my team and I did not stop until we ran out of tests, which fortunately was about the time we were handling the last of the arrivals.

Finally, at day's end, the parking lot empty, a lone car pulled up and the middle-aged man behind the wheel, nodding at the white-haired man sitting next to him, stuck his head out the driver's side window. "My father's been trying to get tested for weeks," he said. An older Black man emerged from the passenger side. "Please test me," he said. "*Please*. The last time I tried I had to leave before they tested me because I had to pick up a body."

Before we could tell him that we were done for the day and could he please come to our next church location a couple days later, he explained that he was a funeral director. All he had been doing every day for weeks was graveside funerals since no one could gather indoors at funeral parlors. A week earlier he was in line to get tested but at the last minute got called away yet again to address another casualty, another human being lost, another body for him to pick up. Afterward, he went home to West Philly and visited one of the university testing sites. They turned him away because he didn't have a prescription from a doctor. The man was old —could they not see that? Couldn't they see that his job was a hazard, not just to him but to others? All the people he was burying had Covid-19. This funeral director was the walking, talking definition of empathy. His eyes had seen too much. Where was the empathy for *him*?

Though we had closed everything down we told him, "Of course we'll test you." We found a couple test kits—I always had a few in reserve—for him and his son, the man behind the wheel. When this seventy-four-year-old Black funeral director, who had been around such constant grief for weeks—way more than even a funeral director is used to—when he saw that we were taking him seriously, he was overcome by tears. Many of us got teary, too.

He was scared. He wanted to be there for the families and help them bury their loved ones. And he also didn't want to go to the hospital and die. We understood that protecting him was also protecting all the people that he was encountering, and all the people *they* were encountering. Testing was not just about helping one individual after another. It was about helping a community, helping the city and the nation as we decreased transmission rates.

Day 1: 12 people tested
Day 2: 150
Day 3: 400
Day 4: 400+
Day 5: 400+

April 26, 2020

Good Day, Dr. Farley,

We are working hard to mitigate the morbidity and mortality associated with COVID19 in the African American communities. To date we have tested over 1,100 residents in 4 days* of testing throughout the city. Our

---

* The total number of residents tested and the number of testing days vary from the totals at the end of the previous section because we had not completed our Day 5 tally when I wrote to the commissioner.

*positivity rate is consistent with percentages from other outpatient testing
sites in Philadelphia and Montgomery County.*

*In line with the recommendations of Dr. Anthony Fauci, National
Institute of Allergy and Infectious Diseases Director, in a meeting
April 25, 2020, with National Academy of Sciences, "the testing efforts
in our country need to double in the weeks coming, to get those infected
with the virus out of the public continuing to transmit the disease." He
also stated that increased testing and resources should be placed in the
African American community where the rates of diagnosis and death
are significantly higher (in a meeting with the Congressional Black
Caucus). Further, White House leadership has called for increased
Mobile testing units. We have acted on ALL recommendations
mentioned above without any city, state or federal financial support.*

*Our testing criteria include: (1) Symptoms consistent with coronavirus
and (2) known exposure to someone positive for coronavirus or presumed
positive. Of note several states have adopted these criteria. A few examples
of patients testing positive by the Black Doctors COVID-19 Consortium
(BDCC) include: (1) a Philadelphia Police Officer, (2) individuals who
tested positive in early April, now asymptomatic, who 3 weeks later are
still positive, (3) several essential employees who were at work when we
called to give them their results, (4) many households where 2 out of 4
family members were unknowingly positive, though they were . . .*

Again, you get the idea. I didn't write Health Commissioner
Thomas Farley to boast of our progress. I wanted him to know that we
were having significant impact and could really use support.

I received the same response I had earlier.

Blah blah blah. Words, no immediate action.

17

WHERE'S THE MONEY?

Over the next several weeks, church leaders in zip codes with some of the highest positivity rates in the city opened their facilities to Black Doctors COVID-19 Consortium and encouraged their congregations and neighboring community to seize the opportunity to test. Women cooked for us so we could have meals. Church members prayed for us. And the people came.

My phone blew up with media requests. Byron's phone, too, with people desperate to get ahold of me. In that dark time, we stood out as an "upbeat" story.

When people working for BDCC asked me who was paying for our operation, I told them straight up: "The money is coming from my pocket and some GoFundMe donations." I didn't say it to brag—to test four hundred people cost around $20,000 a day, for personnel, test processing, and charity care. When I got the inevitable follow-up question, "Dr. Stanford, why doesn't the city give us money?" I also had a stock answer.

"Great question. I'd like to know the same thing."

Area politicians wanted to know more about me. *Is she an ally?*

Can we trust her? Who does she think she is? She won't be around long. I wasn't hiding or playing games. The names of each person we tested were entered into a database that required my national practitioner ID number. All the city Health Department officials had to do was look me up as a licensed Pennsylvania physician to see how many patients we had tested and other information about me. It seemed to take them a while to acknowledge to themselves that, yes, this Dr. Ala Stanford person and this Black Doctors COVID-19 Consortium, whatever the hell that was, were doing something, *now, effectively, innovatively, and legally.*

When it came to government action, it was deaf ears and shrugged shoulders.

Some elected officials thought I would be placated by their referring me to others. It was circular, pointless, maddening. In my conversations with these officials, I was offered things I hadn't asked for and already had, such as the promise of better reimbursement rates with insurance companies. They assumed I had just formed this mom-and-pop business and wasn't already in network with all the major insurance carriers, Medicaid, and Medicare. Or they promised a donation to BDCC but it needed to go through a particular nonprofit . . . which smelled all over the place. I quickly learned that for an organization to allow a donation to us to "pass through" their books, they would want something in return, possibly a little off the top for them, plus the donor of the tax-exempt money would now be in good favor with two organizations. The politicians I was writing didn't know that I had created a nonprofit organization nearly a decade earlier. They also didn't ask.

Or I got a version of this: *Happy to help! . . . now please install our handpicked person to head your little organization.*

Yeah, I was going to do it my way.

My attitude—my transparency and not wanting to play the game— came from a life of being Black in America and having to wait; a life of people telling me and my community, "Not now . . . Be patient . . . Don't worry, help is coming." We at BDCC were doing the work our government was supposed to. This was not our job; not one of us had been doing this before April 16, 2020. But if the government wasn't going to do it, then they could at least provide funding for those of us who were. I hugely salute those that were the beneficiaries of government money, my health care colleagues in hospital ICUs at the time, taking care of the sickest, exposing themselves to enormous risk. For all the credit they got at the time, they deserve so much more.

But my team and I were a front line, too, helping to keep those hospital numbers down, making it easier on the whole stressed system—on ignored neighborhoods, on a fraying health care apparatus, on the city of Philadelphia.

I realized *I* was the action plan I was waiting for. My team was the action plan. Looking back, I understand that the city and state officials who kept rebuffing me were waiting for federal dollars before they could put things into motion—but this was a public health crisis, for crying out loud, this was a local and national and global emergency, where every day that went by without action was more than just one lost day. It was untold numbers of lives.

It was massively frustrating that the city Health Department, hospitals, Federally Qualified Health Centers, all generously funded by the federal government, were inert, dormant, impotent, passive, waiting for their own influx of dollars before anything *out of the ordinary* was done. Philadelphia is known as a city of colleges, universities, medical schools. Some of the world's most prestigious educational institutions and medical systems are located right in those neighborhoods that had high COVID positivity rates. Why were they left to struggle? Shouldn't an out-of-the-ordinary pandemic warrant an out-of-the-ordinary response? When it's a virus we were all fighting, something with no allegiance to anyone or anything? Did these institutions really have *nothing* saved, no discretionary funds they could tap into, to get to the communities with the greatest need? Of *course* there were funds. Of *course* they had liquid cash. I will never accept that I had more money in my bank account than the Philadelphia Department of Public Health.

But they waited for the money. And waited—

Finally! In early May, there was exciting news: The Centers for Disease Control awarded the city of Philadelphia $92 million to be spent over two and a half years for coronavirus testing and contact tracing.[1] Fantastic! The city, in turn, requested proposals from groups that could perform such tests. Great! Beautiful! Who better than us? Mid-May, BDCC submitted a $6.9 million bid.

Meanwhile, our GoFundMe campaign amount approached $50,000; every bit helped. On Mother's Day, Jada Pinkett Smith had me on her Facebook Watch show, *Red Table Talk*, with a few other women, discussing constructive things mothers were doing during the pandemic. At the end of the show, Jada gave me a blessed surprise. "Whatever your GoFundMe total is right now," she said, "the Will and Jada Smith Family Foundation will match it." With their generous support we now had almost $100,000.

But then we got—that is, didn't get—more of the same from the city.

Health Commissioner Farley announced that negotiations were underway with the Public Health Management Corp. and the Philadelphia Mental Health Care Corp., two health care providers that had contracts with the city. By working with organizations that the city "already had established relationships [with] . . . they could circumvent the lengthy competitive bid process required to secure new vendors and get testing underway quickly."[2] Are you serious? Get testing underway quickly? At a city budget meeting in late May, when asked about BDCC's role and our bid for money, Farley replied, "We think [the consortium's work] is great . . . [but] it wasn't like they were the only organization that was offering testing to African Americans."[3]

I'd started this effort out of my own bank account, but without serious money from the city we couldn't go on forever. And insurance companies balked at reimbursing me because I was not an "official" known entity—in this field, who was?—even though as a surgeon I'd been in their network for years. Did my being a Black woman affect my getting paid? I had no proof. I also had no good explanation.

. . .

Nothing surprised me.

So many of our politicians would not have been elected without the support of Black people and the Black church, yet the powers that be were ignoring us, or just not listening. Yes, nobody had ever dealt with anything like this, a public health crisis this complex. But they knew the positive test percentages; at this point, if they didn't, then shame on them. They thought they were helping by opening more testing sites—but you still needed a prescription from a referral doctor. You still had to be a certain age. You still had to have comorbid health conditions. You still needed an appointment during hours that most people were working. If that was the approach, well, more sites did not equal all that much more access.

One day a hospital agreed to cosponsor one of our events. The woman who showed up had a big heart and clearly wanted to help, but she had no support from her own department: She dropped off boxes of chips and other snacks. That was the extent of it.

Reverend Mitchell publicly blasted city leaders. If the mayor's office argued that they were genuinely helping us out (they were not), then the pastor pushed back. He went to war with the city, freeing me to focus on the health care part. It was bad cop, good cop—or, really, bad cop, Florence Nightingale. The media loved our persistence; elected officials didn't know what to do about us. They knew Reverend Mitchell. I remained a largely unknown entity.

To be kind, politicians are generally used to dealing with issues that are not quite so urgent, handling things on the turtle-paced legislative level. Making laws slowly, painstakingly. But this was not about lawmaking. This was about identifying a pressing problem, inaction worsening it by the day, and having the fortitude to make quick, strong decisions. Taking a wait-and-see approach was an insidious, failed strategy. It wasn't a strategy, period.

Meanwhile, Black Doctors COVID-19 Consortium operated like a well-oiled machine. We were getting good, very good, at our process.

Each session, each pop-up church site, we tested hundreds and hundreds. More stories, more tears, more tests, more gratitude. Zip after zip. The volume might have overwhelmed some; for us, the feeling was, *Fine, keep 'em coming. We can handle it.*

My team was more than ready, as long as we had enough test kits. Every person who showed up to work with us was putting in up to twelve hours a day, at times more, knowing that even with PPE and strict protocols they were seriously heightening their own risk of getting Covid-19. We tested people and we comforted people. The members of our team relied on one another for support. Some days I would say to them, "I may seem really crabby and stressed today so I'm going to need you all to lift me up." They always did.

We made our mistakes, like initially promising to call everyone back with their results, positive or negative. The sheer volume made it impossible. I didn't have a fancy electronic medical records system to automatically text results; plus, when someone was positive, they needed medical guidance, contact tracing. They had all kinds of questions. Is a text really adequate?

Eventually, we decided to call only those with a positive diagnosis. Even that was tough, since a 25 percent positivity rate meant roughly one hundred calls per four hundred tests, a number we often hit. For those who tested negative? We finally learned to tell patients that no news was good news. Every so often we diverted from our plan: One woman we tested called repeatedly for days, leaving endless messages on the BDCC voicemail. She was crying. She was talking at lightning speed. She couldn't function until she knew her status. (She came back negative.) But that was the anomaly. I called most of the positives myself so I could talk them through contact tracing. I was on the phone with lots of frightened, anxious people. I hoped my bedside manner was an asset.

One testing day I was informed that someone from the city had stopped by to drop off "supplies": opened boxes of gloves, a size too big to be of much use, and the wrong kind of masks. Useless. The person who came by had announced to one of our staff, *I work for the city, here you go, blah, blah, blah.* My staff member took the boxes, thanked the individual, and asked if they had anything else for Dr. Stanford, to which the person said no. It was clear to my staffer that they were snooping, taking in our operation, presumably to report back to some higher-up. Once, someone dropped off boxes of pens and stress balls with the name of a state senator embossed on them. On more than one occasion people who were obviously not there to get tested started taking photos. (I have no idea if they were with the city or not.) I told them, "Sorry, no pictures, that's a violation, please leave." Suspicious.

My biggest fear was the scarcity of test kits. Since I wasn't a primary care doctor or a hospital, I continually had to push hard for kits, which were difficult to procure. One day, more people than usual showed up, in the rain, and I hated turning them away. But I was fast running out of tests. I called everyone who might have extras. I called every hospital where I'd ever been on staff. Meg McGoldrick, president and CEO of Abington Hospital (my former boss), was the only one who delivered. Businesswoman that she is, she said, "Why don't you just send them to the hospital? We're not far from the church."

"They've been in line already," I said, "plus some of them don't have insurance." I didn't like the idea of asking a mass of people who had been waiting in line to now travel to another place, maybe making them feel as if they were getting jerked around yet again. Our brand was trust, as much as we were providing Covid tests. After a pause, Meg agreed that the best solution was for us to come get test kits from her. I asked Byron to race over to the hospital and pick them up.

That was also the day a film crew for CBS national news came down from New York. I tried to remain calm and upbeat during the interview, but it was another day of crappy weather, and I was quietly freaking out at the prospect of so many people waiting in line with no tests. But Byron arrived just in time with the extra kits—and who knows? Maybe it was a good thing for the world to see how desperate we were simply to have essential supplies.

It's not enough for the powers that be to see a community suffering. If it were, we would never have been in that position. The powers have to hear from that community over and over and over and over until the community's suffering and mistreatment finally influence how those powers make policy. (See also: Flint, Michigan.) Someone once said that those closest to the pain should be closest to the policy; instead, they're often the furthest away. BDCC was the bridge between the policy and the pain.

Individuals took notice that we were in the community not just testing but educating. People posted their experiences with us on social media. News outlets, local and national, began to report on us. Only then did politicians and city officials begin returning our calls.

On a very hot day in early June, back at Enon Tabernacle Baptist Church once again, where BDCC was testing hundreds of people, Philadelphia mayor Jim Kenney and Health Commissioner Thomas Farley held a press conference to announce that Black Doctors COVID-19 Consortium had been awarded a $1.3 million grant. It was less than one-fifth what we had asked for, and actually I shouldn't use the word "grant"; it was technically a "request for funding," which is just like it sounds, slower and more complicated than a grant. But they still wanted to make it public. One politician, hoping to take full advantage of the photo op of the funding announcement, said, "There's never a wrong time to do the right thing," while smiling and waving. If they were being honest, they might have said, "We screwed up, and we've been screwing up since the start of the pandemic. Today is our chance to publicly acknowledge that." The DeSean Jackson Foundation—he of my adored Philadelphia Eagles—also presented a check that day.

Under the hot sun, Mayor Kenney was sweating in his suit; my team and I were in our usual masks, goggles, and PPE. The mayor noted the oppressive weather to me, and the commissioner wondered if we stayed out there in the heat all day? I thought—and didn't say— *Like, how else will people get tested?*

Later, when asked by a reporter what I thought of the financial award, I called it "reasonable."

A week and a half later, at a Juneteenth celebration in West Philly, the mayor came over to me. "My face is still burned from being out there in the heat with you the other day," he said.

We laughed about it. These public displays of support for BDCC by the mayor's office allowed us to bury the hatchet. The city administration could finally see we were among the ones really getting things done and finally began honoring that.

Until they didn't.

We at Black Doctors scheduled a special testing session for funeral directors in the early summer. Close to a hundred people showed up.

Was it really only our small organization that could address such a need in the midst of a pandemic? Why didn't one major health care provider come up with that simple idea? One health insurance company? One state senator or city Health Department administrator? It made perfect sense, for public health and for just being a better human. In a public health crisis, you go to the people.

We were testing five to seven days a week and probably in the news just as often. We didn't call the TV stations. They just showed up, sometimes multiple affiliates and journalists at the same time. It got to the point where I could not watch all the coverage or read all the articles. I was rarely ever home when the six o'clock news came on anyway. What mattered was that attention was being paid.

More great people came to volunteer or take paid positions with us. Some young medical residents who were very busy at hospitals nevertheless found time to volunteer whenever they could squeeze it in. One woman, who had just graduated from nursing school but hadn't yet landed her first job, joined us, staying through the end of the year, when she felt the need to get a hospital job that would challenge her on a wider range of skills. (Eventually she left that for a job with the city Health Department and reported back to me later that at her orientation, page 1 of the manual on Covid testing was essentially the BDCC protocols—exactly what we had learned and recommended.)

The administration went from ignoring us, to observing us, to emulating us, without (of course) crediting us with being initially more effective at managing a public health crisis than they were. As the saying goes: Imitation is the sincerest form of flattery.

I took great pride in what we were doing. There was so much spirit and emotion.

There was the woman who had lost both parents within a day of each other, in tears, wanting to be tested.

There was the young Latina doctor who worked with us, whose eyes were opening to the gross disadvantages in communities of color, telling me how she truly felt that many white people "just aren't getting what we're saying. It's almost like being gaslighted. 'Oh, it's not that bad.' 'It's not that big of a deal.' Yes, it *is* that big of a deal. And the more people that truly see it and understand the disparity, the more we can get help for our families and the rest of the community."

Some testing days, long and complicated and often frustrating, I felt moments of self-pity and thought to myself, *I hope this is over soon so I can go back to surgery full-time and replenish my retirement and my kids' college fund.* Back to my routine of operating two days a week. Back to my comfortable lifestyle. Back to my monthly salary, which would be annual pay for a lot of people. I cringed to consider how much money Byron and I were spending, so I just didn't think about it. When I got home after testing each day, I would go into the garage, strip off my first layer of clothes, and shove them into the wash—decontaminating. I wanted to do more before entering the house, but it's not as if I had a sponge bath out in the garage.

Even with the city award, money and resources were a continuing problem for Black Doctors. It was only after one of the volunteers from my church, a retiree who had worked in the claims department for Independence Blue Cross and Blue Shield, asked if I needed help sorting through all the paperwork (*Yes, please!*) that I started seeing some reimbursement from all I'd laid out. The HRSA (Health Resources and Services Administration), a federal agency, provided a way to be reimbursed for the uninsured.

We at Black Doctors were in a groove, making an impact, but I was also physically and emotionally spent. There had to be a more efficient, effective way to do all this, even with so much uncertainty in the air. A doctor and surgeon by training, I found myself thinking more and more like a health care advocate, like a policy person. I kept thinking how differently I would have acted had *I* been mayor during a public health crisis like Covid.

I would have asked my health commissioner for briefs two to three times daily—or more, as needed.

I would have focused on neighborhoods where the disease predominated. I would have identified a trusted messenger, health care leader, or facility manager in each of these zips, then partnered with the leaders of a prominent organization in the community. I would have compensated these leaders for their input.

I would have determined which groups were most affected—grocery clerks, bus drivers, etc.

I would have used hotels and dormitories immediately to separate the infected. (The current way was for hospitals to tell those infected to stay away from them and others, without giving them a place to go.)

I would have used emergency funds for all the city's major hospitals to set up testing locations outside in their parking lots, removed barriers such as requirements for referrals and insurance, and ensured that test sites were open on nights and weekends.

I would have called on all FQHCs to have longer hours, not shorter, while making sure they had adequate PPE and rotating staff (the latter, to decrease burnout as well as exposure to the virus). Too many health care workers were sheltering in place; too many FQHCs were closed early and/or accepted only those enrolled with them.

I would *not* have waited for the CARES (Coronavirus Aid, Relief, and Economic Security) Act to be passed to get started.

I would have gone around the city to see for myself what trends were unfolding. By identifying the groups that were most affected, I would not have unintentionally favored one group over another.

Easy to say, I know. But that's what I would have done. And it's not as if anything I was asking for was impossible.

The August 2020 issue of *Pediatrics* published an article titled "Race, Postoperative Complications, and Death in Apparently Healthy Children," which compared health outcomes for healthy Black children and white children after basic procedures; it found that the former suffered significantly more post-operative hospitalizations and deaths. Many of us had been talking about this for years, but the response was often disbelief or outright doubt about the research, reminiscent of my colleague's reaction when I presented the paper on the poorer health outcomes of Hispanic children versus white children after midgut volvulus operations. Now, with the inherently, if covertly, biased response to Covid-19, I hoped that studies like the one published in *Pediatrics* would open people's eyes.

By late summer of 2020, BDCC and the city had made great progress in testing underserved neighborhoods, and I considered leaving my role and heading back to the OR . . . but then autumn came, and what happened? Lots of kids returned to school, including colleges, started living together again in dorms, having parties after a half-year of isolating and Zooming at home . . . and a new strain of Covid-19 spread, sending the positive rates back up. We had more work to do.

In October, when the president got infected with Covid, it was another slap in the face to so many of the people in my community— not that anyone expected the president of the United States to get less than the very best medical care. But it was obvious that, as one of my colleagues said, "no one's getting the treatment 45's getting." He didn't mean the round-the-clock care at Walter Reed National Military Medical Center that 45 was entitled to, but access to medication like a high IV dose of remdesivir, or an antibody drug from Regeneron that was experimental at the time, or the steroid dexamethasone, reserved for a privileged few.

As 45 improved, he had the nerve to proclaim about the virus: "Don't worry about it." I understood it was necessary to keep people from panicking. But to say "don't worry" when you're one of the tiny, very privileged few to receive intravenous doses of drugs that are experimental or in limited supply? What a selfish, tin-eared statement. Hospitalized folks with Covid, including friends of mine and the spouse of one of my BDCC nurses, did not have access to these medications. I heard about a state senator who got Covid and was given the special antibody cocktail; I heard the same about another local politician. So, as always, if you knew someone who knew someone, you got special treatment. It wasn't anything that shocked those in my community. They—we—knew all too well that outcomes and opportunities are so often not created equal. But now, in a life-and-death struggle with a virus whose infectiousness spared few, the gross inequality in access and care was a bitter pill to swallow. Or maybe it was a pill that only some people got to swallow.

The infection, hospitalization, and death rates for Blacks in the U.S. were still distressingly elevated, three times higher than those for white people.[4] As Pastor Mitchell said, "This is no longer benign neglect. This is malignant neglect." He was right. We knew exactly where the most impacted lived, knew their zip codes, their ethnicity. We knew, as we've always known.

Toward the end of the year, after months and months of our testing success, Mayor Kenney shared that the way that BDCC approached the problem—Black people needed extra, barrier-free access to testing—had been right. Kenney acknowledged the bias against BDCC and publicly stated that the city did not get it right in the beginning. The admission didn't benefit the people who had needed those resources earlier, but hopefully it would help as we moved forward. (Eventually we received the mayor's Magis Award for community service, handed to me by Mayor Kenney.)

In December we learned that the first vaccines for Covid—medicine that would diminish the virus's infectiousness and, for those infected, blunt its severity—would be available very soon, remarkably so. The mRNA vaccines from Moderna and Pfizer and the viral vector vaccine from Johnson & Johnson were about to be approved under Emergency Use Authorization, which the Food and Drug Administration could invoke during a public health emergency.

I hoped vaccinating would proceed more equitably than testing.

18

MOVING THE NEEDLE

Trust is not a light switch you can flip on or off. It takes time to develop.

When we started to vaccinate in early 2021, folks in their eighties and nineties—even the occasional hundred-year-old—came to our sites very wary. *Is this for Black people? Why is your operation just for Black people?* Seeing that my PPE-garbed associates and I were Black wasn't enough to ease their suspicions. Black folks of a certain age were justified in associating Black-directed medical campaigns with the notorious Tuskegee study, or maybe the exploitation of Henrietta Lacks. Maybe they worried that this was just the latest version of strangers trying to convince them to put something in their body supposedly to help, but instead causing harm. They weren't buying it, not at first. The long, tainted history of the mistreatment of Blacks by the American medical system had caused so many of us, for generations, to lack basic trust in anyone in a health care setting. How would we at Black Doctors get past all that? How would we get people to *want* to get vaccinated?

Trust was essential to make BDCC's transition from testing to vaccinating successful. It helped that we had developed trust by Covid-testing communities basically in their backyards, five to seven days a week, beginning in April 2020. It was now January 2021, and we were still out there. We didn't cut and run. We didn't take a photo op and wipe our hands and move on. We had stayed, week after week, month after month, working hard to get the job done, to bring the numbers down. We were just about the only ones doing it consistently for this particular, neglected, sizable population. We were there for people who were genuinely sick. We were medically competent and emotionally available. When positivity rates decreased and the funding for other testing entities stopped, they immediately closed up shop. Few of them reopened. We never went away.

We had gotten good at testing as many as eight hundred people a day, but vaccinating would be more complicated. We had to be approved as a community vaccination partner. Medical oversight of the administration of shots had to be performed by a licensed vaccinator, done in a way consistent with standards of medical care. We had to agree to adhere to the Covid-19 community vaccination program requirements of the city of Philadelphia. We would need enough doses, syringes, freezers, refrigerators, alcohol, Band-Aids.

I'm proud that the community trusted us; I'm proud of the work we did to earn that trust. But did they trust America enough to take the vaccine? Did they trust Big Pharma, which had come up with it? If enough people of color refused a vaccine that would very likely do much more good than harm, for them individually and certainly for the community, then *why* was that?

Before I could fully answer that last question, I had another question that needed answering, one that could impact those around me, both staff and community members:

Was *I* going to get vaccinated?

One day back in August of 2020 I felt unwell and had Judge Greg Scott, a volunteer, drive me home from a church testing site. I was feverish and tired, but my first Covid test came back negative. I stayed in our guest bedroom for several days. My kids brought food to the door. (There are upsides to illness.) I slept a lot. I had my doctor's bag nearby, pulse oximeter, blood pressure cuff, stethoscope. I had acetaminophen. I did my own vitals, took my temperature. I didn't reach oxygen levels that were dangerously low. I was just very achy and tired—and scared. At one point, I felt so crappy, I hallucinated I was going to die. I reviewed my will. Back then it took about two days for a PCR test (polymerase chain reaction, a more definitive test) to come back, and by the time my result returned, also negative, I felt better. Maybe I hadn't gotten Covid after all.

Two months later, in the fall, at my doctor's for an annual wellness check, I discovered that I had Covid-19 antibodies. So I *had* been infected! Likely it was that awful bout in August. I was actually relieved; now I wouldn't have to get the vaccine that was coming out soon—at least not immediately.

But then people, including my staff, began to ask me, "Are you getting the shot?"

When I told them I wasn't because I had been infected and had antibodies, they respected that . . . but then quite a few of them told me that if I wasn't taking it, then they weren't. That didn't make much medical sense—they didn't have antibodies and I did—but, again: trust. Word spread. A number of my church members told me, more or less, "When you tell me to roll up my sleeve, Doc, I will." *If it's good enough for you, it's good enough for me.* Never mind the sound reasoning for my not getting it right away: To others, the fact that I wasn't taking it meant it wasn't good enough for me.

As a leader whom others trusted with their own medical decisions, I was torn. Initially, I *did* have reservations about the vaccine. I thought it might have been authorized and distributed for use too soon. I knew that no vaccine had ever been developed in under four years. I knew that the federal government's impressive Operation Warp Speed had concentrated their efforts and those of Big Pharma like maybe nothing before, but I also knew that Pfizer and Moderna were not the companies that had led the way in previous vaccine development; that had been Merck, GlaxoSmithKline, Sanofi, and others. Even had those latter companies led the charge, I don't know that I would have been confident in *any* vaccine developed at such lightning speed.

To be clear: I was not categorically antivaccine. My sons got the HPV vaccine, one of the most recent vaccines. All the kids had gotten the chickenpox vaccine. But there was a track record with that. There was no track record for the Covid vaccine.

Before I was a doctor, before I was a surgeon, I was a Black woman. And I was raised to believe that you go to the doctor only when you're really sick or you think you're about to die. The past experiences of countless Black people taught us to be wary, if not fearful.

Science Ala was reading the transcript from the FDA's Emergency Use Authorization hearing and every other medical-scientific-technical report she could get her hands on.

Black Ala wasn't sure she was gonna do this.

For Science Ala, taking the Covid vaccine made sense. For Black Ala, the report wasn't totally convincing. You could spin the evidence either way. On one hand, clinical trials had shown amazing effectiveness and remarkably few side effects, plus research and testing on messenger RNA, or mRNA, the type of vaccine Moderna and Pfizer were dispensing, had been going on for decades. On the other hand, too little time had passed for us to know about potential longer-term side effects in humans.

I had gone to my doctor every four weeks to have my antibodies checked; we had agreed that I didn't need to get the vaccine until IgG antibodies were no longer present.

But then the vaccination question—*Will she or won't she?*— became real, and I had to take a stand. It became less about me and more about all those around me getting infected and dying at a rate greater than any cohort in the country. *They* couldn't get their antibodies checked every four weeks like I could. Following my doctor's advice might have been right for me as an individual, but not for the masses of people we were trying to serve and protect. They needed validators, people in the community who they considered trusted health care providers.

So, yeah, forget what *I* thought. It was a time for thinking about our neighbors, not just ourselves. That wasn't easy, especially in American society, where we're taught to be individuals, often to an extreme that's harmful for community and society and that, in the end, sometimes backfires on us as individuals. For way too many people, it was every man and woman for themselves. The national mentality was survival of the fittest.

I realized how important it was for me to be open and honest and encouraging with all those who looked to me for guidance on the vaccine. I knew how important it was to push for its widespread adoption, but I also made it a point to listen, really listen, to each person's reason for skepticism. I was there to educate, not convince. There were many reasons for hesitation, some more valid than others. One woman told me that because she had had an allergic reaction to hair dye, she thought she was allergic to vaccines. I told her that was untrue. Several people told me that they were avoiding the vaccine because they were immunocompromised; I explained that that was precisely why they *should* get vaccinated.

More and more test-takers asked me my stance on the vaccine— especially now that we had started to provide flu shots at each test stop, too—so we put together a BDCC survey (a psychometric tool) to assess attitudes and perceptions of our patients.

"Do you think the vaccine will make you sick?"

Most answered no.

"Do you think the vaccine will be approved without adequate safety measures?"

Most worried yes.

"Do you plan to get it as soon as it becomes available?"

More said no than yes.

"Do you trust the government to deliver a safe and effective vaccine to your community?

More answered yes than no, but only slightly.

"Do you think drug companies are producing vaccines that may harm your community?"

More than twice as many said no than yes.

"Will you get vaccinated only at your primary care doctor?"

Slightly more than half said no.

The questionnaire surveyed 583 people—87 percent African American, 10 percent white, 3 percent Hispanic. Females made up 56 percent of the respondents. Eighty-six percent of those who answered had insurance.

The dangers of the disease seemed to outweigh suspicions about the vaccine—not by a lot but enough. Since we were doing our work in church parking lots, we could see a funeral happening almost every day, often more than one. Even the skeptics had to pause and consider what we were there for, and had they really taken every reasonable precaution against this enemy?

With the vaccine authorization date imminent, Byron said he was going to take it. The kids, not yet eligible, were all, *No way, no how*, which didn't surprise me (kids think they're invincible and don't particularly like needles). The chance of children and young people getting severely sick from Covid was extremely small, unless you were a child of color.[1]

After another day of leading my team at a mobile testing site, I stopped on my way home to see my pastor. "Are you going to get vaccinated?" I asked.

"What do you think I should do?" he asked.

"I don't know," I said, which I'm sure he didn't find helpful.

"Whatever you tell me to do, Ala, I'll do."

When I got home, I felt torn. I cried in the shower. The next morning, I knew. I shared it with my husband. I informed Pastor Mitchell that yes, I was getting the vaccine. I told my staff the same. Ultimately, my team and I made a collective decision to get vaxxed publicly, together. It was important that the people around me, and those who looked to me for guidance, see that I was getting it. Covid-19 forced everyone to say, *It's not just about me but the person next to me.* At least, that's what it *should* have made us say.

On Wednesday, December 16, 2020, as a snowstorm blanketed the city, most of my staff, close to twenty of us, went down to the Health Department and got vaccinated. It was pretty emotional.

I had a terrible reaction to my shot. Byron had no reaction to his.

Yes, the vaccine was good enough for me, because it had to be good enough for others.

Two weeks later, on the last day of the historic year of 2020, New Year's Eve, my birthday, I reserved a suite at the Four Seasons to celebrate with Byron. We had so much to be thankful for. But then it turned out that a staff member at one of Byron's companies tested positive, and they had shared a car ride; we were between shots and not yet optimally protected, so he had to quarantine—away from me and the kids. I spent the night alone, in a beautiful hotel suite, ordering room service and watching the fireworks and the clock strike midnight by myself.

Given the rare occasion to take a few breaths and reflect on my life, I realized something fundamental: While I was trained as a surgeon, my goal from the very beginning of my love affair with medicine was to provide what was needed to the most vulnerable communities, which happened to be the one I came from. My training, combined with my pride in and love for Black people, was designed to let me serve. And serve we did, where the need was greatest. You have to give people what they need, where they are, how they are.

I had been called. By my city. By my people. By my own.

FALSE NARRATIVE, REAL SCAM

"Black people don't want the vaccine."

That was the response from a woman at the Philadelphia Department of Public Health, when I called to tell them that we at BDCC were set up and ready to administer the vaccine as soon as it was available.

"We can't afford to waste it when other people want it more," she added.

That was the narrative. *Other people.* It was misleading, as our own survey had shown. Yes, there was skepticism among Blacks (and among other people of color, and among whites, too), but a significant and growing number of African Americans were as eager as anyone to get vaccinated, and many were desperate. I asked to be allowed to start vaxxing that month, January 2021, but the earliest the city would agree to was some vague time in February. We couldn't start until then, I was informed, because BDCC was "not ready." What the hell did that mean? When I pushed them on it, they admitted unapologetically to the real reason for the delay:

"Black people are hesitant . . . They don't want it . . . We can't waste it on them . . . We don't have enough."

A destructive myth.

Was it true that African Americans, who made up over 40 percent of the population of Philadelphia, represented a far smaller percent of those vaccinated so far? Yes. Was it true that vaccine uptake among health care workers—the cohort being vaxxed most in those first weeks—was much lower for those of color than white health care workers? Also yes. But there were significant reasons for those disparities. "Black people are hesitant" and "Black people don't want it" were generalizations and not universally true.

I referenced my objective survey data. "This is what I've been doing as a physician-scientist," I told the keepers of the vaccine. "We have the information!" It would take too long to get the study into a legitimate scientific journal, and time mattered. I had to spread the word myself. And the part of my survey that appeared to feed their narrative—documented hesitation on the part of Black people—mostly had to do with *who* was administering the vaccine.

I would prove the level of interest another way. My team created an online portal; the venue bothered me a bit because it could be accessed only by people with an internet connection, narrowing the audience. Still, within forty-eight hours of the portal's going live, thousands had signed up for the vaccine—and our analytics told us that *over 95 percent of the signees were Black*. We had the interest! And since we at Black Doctors were old hands at mass Covid testing, we could handle mass Covid vaccination, despite what some authority figures may have thought. All we needed were doses and, crucially, an official go-ahead from the city.*

---

* The reason I took so much issue with my city of Philadelphia and not with my state of Pennsylvania: Philly was one of several American cities receiving a direct vaccine allotment from the CDC, without its passing through the state.

As we fought for authorization, I paid close attention to the way vaccination for the general population was being mapped out. I was disturbed to see that everything seemed to be "by appointment." By now it's probably obvious why this upset me: Appointments were available only during the day, while most people—many of them people of color—couldn't easily take off of work.

While we waited, I heard on the news of an upcoming mass vaccination event in Philadelphia. It was odd to learn of it that way, given what I'd been involved in for months, given my growing network—and given that I was on the Department of Health Covid response team. But how could I complain about such a development? It sounded like a good thing, so long as it was done the right way. And it seemed to be. The group to be vaccinated was more health care workers who, heaven knows, needed and deserved early protection. I just hoped that "health care workers" also included those at hospitals and other medical facilities who transported patients, who brought patients food, who emptied the garbage, who worked security in the ER, and others like them. Those folks were often just as exposed to the virus as doctors and nurses, and they were predominantly people of color. So many of the health care workers who had died of Covid so far were people of color, mostly Black and Asian/Pacific Islander.[1]

Then I read that an organization named Philly Fighting COVID had been awarded a contract from the city of Philadelphia for nearly a million dollars to vaccinate citizens. They were the ones running the mass vaccination. For months I had been hearing about PFC running testing clinics, and almost nothing about the organization impressed me. They were led by a twenty-two-year-old Drexel graduate student with no medical experience. The leadership didn't hide their youth and inexperience but rather boasted about it: In media coverage, the founder referred to Philly Fighting COVID as "a bunch of kids" (*New York Times*) and "college kids" (*Philadelphia Inquirer*).[2] Though they had been contracted to test underserved communities, they kept shoddy records on patients. They had collected data from fewer than one-third of those they tested, more than two-thirds of whom were white. In the days leading up to and following the big vaccination event, more dirt was rumored or exposed. They had supposedly been taking vaccines home with them. They had tested City Council people in their homes. There were people on the organization's payroll who didn't show up to work. They allegedly sold to third parties the personal data of people who had signed up for vaccination. They had quietly switched from being a nonprofit organization to a for-profit.

Here we at BDCC were, doing the work . . . and the city shows a greater comfort level with them than us? The words "systemic, institutionalized bias" can be used often enough that they start losing their meaning, yet this development—a largely unvetted organization run by a young white entrepreneur gets a whole bunch of money, while Black Doctors keeps begging for it—seemed like the poster child for such thinking. Had the city really seen *no* red flags before they partnered with these people? Did they do *any* due diligence?

In my mind, Philly Fighting COVID were grifters that lacked integrity who had seen what we at BDCC had been doing with testing, the incredibly positive media coverage we received, and they seized on a desperate moment and a desperate town. They recognized an easy opportunity to grab city funds. Just market themselves as a supposedly competent, nongovernment, entrepreneurial alternative providing an essential, assembly-line service in a city that appeared to have no clue what it was doing.

One large difference between us and Philly Fighting COVID was that we did our work *before* there was money being handed out. *Before* someone asked. We did it as soon as we recognized that underserved people were not being adequately cared for and we could do something about it, not *after* it appeared to be a great for-profit enterprise. We kept records on everyone we tested. We tested the underserved people we had promised to test.

Philly Fighting COVID wasn't the only one going after the money.

The administration at a large local hospital invited Black Doctors to join them in their effort to vaccinate the underserved Black and brown population because there was a FEMA (Federal Emergency Management Agency) grant waiting for hospitals who could show that they were focusing on the most vulnerable, disproportionally impacted populations. I could see that they just wanted to use me. BDCC didn't have access to the grant, but we knew how to find the people. They gave us a negligible fee. I found some comfort in knowing that people were getting serviced. Meanwhile, for me it was a weekly struggle to pay my staff.

The week before Rev. Dr. Martin Luther King Jr. Day of Service, my phone rang. Philly Fighting COVID had been tapped to provide vaccination for a big event that day, but they wouldn't be there. A Black community was once again being left out to dry. "Could you do a vax clinic on MLK Day?" the Health Department woman asked. It was the same person who had told me not very long ago that BDCC could not start vaccinating until February. That we weren't "ready."

"But you told me we needed to wait," I replied innocently.

Something did not smell right.

I was not going to clean up the mess of the Philadelphia Department of Public Health and Philly Fighting COVID. We declined to participate; besides, we already had a big testing event planned for that day, at Girard College.

Sure enough, forty-eight hours later, I learned that the Department of Public Health was canceling their contract with PFC. Details were slowly leaking out. In a subsequent investigation into the mess, the city's inspector general reported that the department had "conducted very little independent research on the applications" for those administering testing; vetting rose to the level of "simple Google searches." Question: Why didn't BDCC's work impress them while they were googling? Beats me. After the dissolution became public, I had a very heated conversation with Health Commissioner Farley about it; by the end of the week, the Health Department delivered one thousand vaccine doses to us for our first vaccination events. I posted a video online announcing locations, dates, and times. We took people in the order they had signed up on our portal.

By 7 a.m. on Saturday, January 16, the line of folks bundled up in parkas, ski pants, hats, gloves, and scarves stretched around the block. We weren't starting until ten.

Five hundred shots in arms. It was an effective first day, much better than our first day of testing, when we went door to door and managed to test all of twelve people.

On Sunday we vaccinated another five hundred people.

We were given more doses. On Monday, MLK Jr. Day, we vaccinated hundreds more. I roamed the site, not only to be seen but also because we were averaging at least a few people passing out per day. It wasn't the vaccine itself that caused people to faint. More likely it was the waiting in line coupled with the stress of getting the shot that overwhelmed them. Dehydration or hypoglycemia or other health problems also contributed. I couldn't help but feel that each case was an example of what happens when people go too long without attention.

Now that the city had officially severed ties with Philly Fighting COVID, we were also receiving all the people who had registered with them, including those who got their first shot with PFC. My organization was getting twice the volume. And still standing.

Early February we were vaccinating inside Fellowship Hall (formerly the gym at Deliverance Evangelistic Church) in North Philadelphia. It was too cold to be outside vaccinating. Every so often, I would stop administering shots and walk the line to see how everyone was doing, make sure the older people were okay. Looking out the window I noticed several particularly nice cars, out of place for North Philly; I also noticed, in line, six young white people of college age. I didn't want to express anger, but I felt it. We had promoted a list of medical conditions provided by the Department of Health—hypertension, diabetes, obesity, cardiovascular disease, asthma—that put you on the list for getting a shot. Apparently, they were all asthmatic.

"All six of you?" I asked.

They nodded. Only one of them could prove it—she not only had an inhaler but a prescription with her name on it—but here they were putting me in the position of turning away people claiming they suffered from a medical condition that placed them at increased risk of having severe disease with Covid-19. It's not as if I had an infinite supply of vaccine. I recognized I needed to address this before it got out of hand.

"The public-facing workers who are more susceptible to contracting and transmitting Covid are the ones who need it most," I told the six of them. "They're helping to keep this country running and have far less access to it." These people were not helping the public health emergency by getting vaxxed in this neighborhood and then going back to the suburbs where they were sheltering in place and working from home. We vaccinated them.

Carpetbagging was happening all over the city and country, and Philadelphia was no exception. Those who had jobs where they were either already working from home or otherwise had enough flexibility to get vaxxed somewhere at ten in the morning, did so. They drove in from the suburbs, BMWs, Range Rovers, Teslas, probably from wealthy Bucks County or maybe affluent Montgomery County. Most people in our community arrived by subway, bus, or foot. There were reports from around the country that rich folks, mostly white, were going into poor neighborhoods, mostly Black and brown, to get vaccinated.

Within forty-eight hours of my encounter with the six students, I created a zip code list, instructing my team from now on to verify that people in line were from the high-risk communities I had identified.

We began checking documents showing proof of residence. I made it clear to all that if you didn't live in a neighborhood that was disproportionately impacted, you would not be vaccinated, at least not by us. Some people showed up with a deed for a building in the neighborhood.

"But do you *live* here?" I asked.

They just angrily pushed the deed in my face.

Other ineligibles got belligerent with my staff, insisting that they get vaccinated, that they had every right, that this was discriminatory . . . it was a bad look. For them. I know that people were crazy during the peak of Covid—Black, white, brown, every shade, all of us—but exerting privilege was ugly. I caught a lot of Twitter flak. Hate mail.

"How dare she do that with government funds?!"

"Can you believe what she's doing with your taxpayer dollar?"

"She's refusing to vaccinate citizens!"

Months before I had been invited to join the city's Vaccine Advisory Committee (VAC), which set priorities for vaccine-eligible populations based on the recommendations of a similar federal committee; I sat on the Committee for Racial Inclusion and Equity, which was folded into the VAC to rectify disparity.

There I was, sitting in committee meetings, listening to plans for rolling out vaccines. Yet in a city that was 44 percent Black, just 12 percent of total vaccinations had gone into Black arms.[3]

It wasn't old-style racism that accounted for this. The city officials in charge of dispensing vaccines didn't hate Black people. The fundamental issue was that people in power remained blind to the lived reality of Black Americans.

What did vaccine expansion and rollout mean to the committees? "Digital registration" for appointments through "your WiFi" or "your phone app." It sounded like Silicon Valley's version of efficiency. It was modern. It was high-tech. Appointments were available at particular sites during particular hours during the daytime. Many African Americans have smartphones, of course, but so many of those in the neighborhoods we were serving lacked unlimited data, or an internet connection at home, or the bandwidth to complete the registration forms for the mandatory appointments during hours when most work. "By appointment only" was part of a larger stuck mindset. The mayor and the health commissioner were preaching concern—"We've got to reach those communities," they said, more or less—but their actions said something else.

It's only health equity *when it results in action*. Authorities could use all the right buzzwords and phrases—"trauma-informed care," "cultural competence," "cultural humility," "safe space" . . . Hello, Philadelphia? What is your health equity *action plan*?

Even after the success of BDCC's testing program and all the lessons it offered, officialdom was making some of the same mistakes with the vaccines. They listened to technocrats. They had hired an inexperienced, corrupt team to administer vaccines, while passing over those of us who'd been on the ground.

Meet people where they live, how they live, when they live. Hadn't our mobile Covid-19 testing program shown that, by coming to Black church parking lots, locations the community knew and trusted, it was possible to make an anxiety-filled experience more convenient and palatable *for the people "we've got to reach"*?

Yet here we were, in the next major phase of the pandemic, doing the exact opposite of what we'd demonstrated actually worked for Black communities. Of *course* the vast majority of the vaccines went to white people! There was no targeted marketing by the city to the most impacted, at-risk Black communities. The city had done it for seniors, hadn't they? Why not for Black folks?

For the last week of February we planned our most ambitious endeavor yet: a twenty-four-hour vaccination marathon to be held at the Liacouras Center at Temple University. Why not? As a surgical intern, resident surgeon, and attending surgeon, I'd often worked twenty-four hours in a row, so why not twenty-four hours of this? To be eligible, patients had to be from one of the Philly zip codes at highest risk for infection, hospitalization, and death; we also looked to vax the elderly and those with chronic conditions. The line for a shot started forming by 9 a.m., in a growing snowstorm. We had folding chairs. We asked everyone to dress warm and be patient: They did, and they were. Some people waited as long as seven hours, but seemed pleased with how they were treated. When the twenty-four hours were up, we had vaccinated four thousand people, hundreds more than the entire city of Philadelphia did in a typical day.

"I don't know too much about how Philadelphia has handled it," said one of the people we vaccinated during the event, "but I know how the Black Doctors have handled it."

A few days later the city policy changed. They announced they were going to "oversample" from zip codes with high poverty rates, which is exactly what we were already doing. They began checking IDs and residency, turning away the well-to-do suburbanites in Range Rovers who were trying to jump the long, long line of folks.

It hardly felt like victory. The news reported that "residents of dozens of suburban zip codes are being vaccinated using city supply at rates almost four times that of the least vaccinated areas of Philadelphia." More than 40 percent of Philly's first vaccination doses, which were supposed to go to city residents, went to those living outside the city.[4] This could be explained, according to Health Commissioner Farley, because lots of health care workers and first responders who worked in Philadelphia lived outside the city limits. But one of his department's spokespeople admitted that vaccine providers, relying mostly on the honor system, had done an inadequate job of vaxxing city residents.

Black vaccination percentages finally started to rise. The last week of February, 22 percent of Philadelphians vaccinated were African American.[5] That felt like a small victory.

Two days later, the last day of the month, I appeared on *Good Morning America*, highlighting the work BDCC was doing. The texts and voicemails and emails that followed were incredibly positive.

For the most part.

Its great what you're doing, working hard to get people vaccinated. But you need a vaccine for all those lazy Black people sitting around doing nothing but collecting welfare checks. That's what you need. Because that's who they all are. But not you.

20

MEET THE NEED

Proximity was critical. As with testing, our vaxxing numbers were impressive because we were right there in the community, with people able to get to us easily, on their own schedule, using their own mode of transportation. By being situated right in their neighborhood, sometimes for several days, we gained something else: We were being *seen* by people who might otherwise have been suspicious of what we were doing, or wary of *anyone* doing what we were doing. (For some folks, our being Black wasn't enough to tip the scales into trust.) From behind the windows of public housing units, from inside a McDonald's, from their porches, people could see Black and brown doctors and health care professionals (and some white ones, too) running a smooth, competent operation—a consistent, reliable presence—allowing many of these observers to make that last mental leap they needed to get vaccinated. Lots of people came by, dipping their toe in the water.

"So . . . you vaccinated?" I asked one man observing the whole operation with great curiosity.

"Nah, not gettin' that, Doc. I appreciate what you're doin' but that ain't for me."

But we returned to that spot again that week and so did the skeptics, and after they'd seen hundreds of people go through the process, including people they may have known, and so many people who looked like them, their objections began to melt. They were in. Some just wanted to get it over with. "No, I don't want to talk about shit, just give me the shot." Some were just waiting for us to charge them some hidden fee—"You know, I can't pay, I gotta get birthday gifts for my daughter." We never charged, of course. We were keeping promises, not breaking them.

There were those whose antivax stance was hard to understand. One day, my operations person brought a LabCorp employee over to me. I recognized him because he picked up our PCR specimens every day.

"He's not vaccinated," said Troy, my ops guy, before leaving us alone.

"So let me get this straight," I said to the LabCorp fellow, trying not to lecture or belittle. "All day long you're picking up specimens of people, many of whom have Covid."

"Yep," he said.

"And you're not vaccinated?"

He started telling me about how he had read a lot, he was interested in the vaccine, but it was still early—

"Seriously, man, hasn't it been long enough? Millions of people have gotten the vaccine, with remarkably few serious issues. I'm vaxxed. Back in December. You've had time to watch us. I'm not dead. I don't have horns growing out of my head. I didn't have a seizure. You know what else I don't have?"

"What?"

"Covid."

He ended up getting vaccinated the next day.

I talked with people about how exactly their religious beliefs precluded their getting vaccinated. Some Catholics, and some who were not Catholic, objected because they thought the vaccine used fetal cells or tissue, which was untrue. I pointed out that the Pope was fully vaxxed. Some Muslims I spoke with said they were unwilling to put anything impure in their bodies; on the other hand, we had entire Muslim families come to get vaccinated. The DoorDash delivery guy who brought me my Sweetgreen order one day, his mask pulled down carelessly over his chin, told me he was washed in the blood of Jesus; it was that, not a vaccine, that would save him.

"What if I told you that I believe that Jesus has put me here to protect *you*," I said, "and to tell you to wear your mask correctly?"

"I know your guys' thing and I'm not getting the shot," he said. "I'll only get it if I have to for work." He looked me up and down, then said, "Damn, you're a doctor. Are you married?"

"Thanks for my food," I said. "Pull your mask up," I scolded him.

It was conversations like that that made us stay in locations multiple days. It could take a while to win people over.

Wherever we went, we rarely had excess vaccines at the end of the day. My team had become expert at knowing how many doses to prepare and how to deliver them efficiently. It was remarkable how good they'd become at all aspects of the operation; any Fortune 500 company would have been lucky to have my people working for them. Late each day, when we calculated that we might have some leftover vaccine, we called around to see who wanted what remained. One of the people we reached asked which type. "Is it the Black one?"

"The Black one?" my staff member responded.

Because there are so many Black people named Johnson, the man on the phone thought the Johnson & Johnson shot was designed specifically for Blacks. "I'll take any vaccine but the Black one," he said.

One day in early March we vaccinated across the street from a big funeral home, one of those massive, banquet hall–sized parlors that can host four funerals simultaneously without anyone knowing the others are going on. That was sad. What was sadder was having so many people stuffed into airless rooms, perhaps beyond capacity, especially at funerals for people dead of Covid. And lots of attendees *still* weren't wearing masks. It was a classic superspreader event. I crossed the street wearing my North Face jacket embroidered with my name and my

Black Doctors COVID-19 Consortium ID. It made me look official but not menacing. I was wearing my mask, of course. I "wandered" into the funeral home, observing people packed like sardines into chapels and waiting rooms. I don't know to whom I said the first words out of my mouth—"Are you serious?" Maybe to a funeral parlor employee. Maybe a funeral attendee. Probably myself.

I crossed back to our vaxxing site, asked one of my staff to run off some flyers, and ten minutes later I was back inside the funeral parlor, clutching dozens of handouts promoting the locations and dates of our next several vax events.

"How you guys doing?" I said to one of the funeral parlor employees.

"Okay," he said, nodding toward the nearest of the overflowing chapels. "Another one from Covid."

"Listen, do you think anyone here wants to get vaccinated? We're right across the street."

Several men who drove hearses and other family cars jumped at the chance. We rushed them across the street and were able to give them shots before the funerals were finished. "Can you speed it up a little?" said one driver, tapping his foot, nervous he was going to be late. "I gotta get back to the car." I made sure to get my little speech to the men—how they still needed a second shot; how they weren't fully protected for at least another few weeks; how they should still use precautions—and sent them on their way.

Then I handed out flyers—not to the funeral home workers but directly to mourners on their way to their cars. If they didn't count as a receptive audience, then no one did.

When I'd run out of flyers, I just talked real talk with some of the funeral home employees. I sensed they wanted an ear. They talked about how tough it had been with so many deaths from Covid. "You know that a corpse can still transmit coronavirus, right?" I said. "And you're dressing it and everything. Are you guys vaccinated?"

"We know, Doc, we know," one of them said.

"Come on, we're right here. Across the street. We've made it easy."

I used my voice to point out the obvious, and they listened.

March 12, 2021, we started vaccinating in homes for those who couldn't easily get out, mostly the elderly. On March 14, we hit an incredible milestone: Black Doctors COVID-19 Consortium had vaccinated 25,000 Philadelphians. Our communities were getting more and more knowledgeable about what they needed to do to protect themselves. We continued seeking out the overlooked.

On a day in mid-April I visited the notorious K&A, Kensington and Allegheny, also known as The Badlands, perhaps the most dangerous, entrenched IV drug–using community in America. I was there to try and vaccinate some of the residents, a tall task. A woman in her sixties with track marks on her arm smoked a crack pipe while we conversed. A medical student who had accompanied us was recording our encounter on her phone. I mentioned the types of Covid vaccines available. In this particular case, I recommended the one-shot J&J, which had just been reauthorized after a brief suspension because of an extremely rare side effect; this woman had housing insecurity, no phone, and no computer access, so it would be hard to locate her for a second shot. She took another drag on the pipe. "Oh, you're not giving me the Johnson & Johnson," she said. "That shit'll kill you"—then she promptly turned to the student to tell her to stop recording, since the student had not obtained proper consent. I smiled—another example of someone so easy to underestimate. This woman was obviously very smart, and knowledgeable about the pandemic. Her struggle with addiction didn't change that.

Communities of color needed us more than ever, but I realized I'd come to a fork in my own road. I was still taking calls in my private practice. The hospital wanted me to continue doing emergency surgery. I'd worked all my adult life to reach the point of being an in-demand, well-regarded pediatric surgeon. Now, though, it had become obvious that I couldn't do it all. I was stretched thin. I had started something important, to me and to the underserved of Philadelphia, and through the determination of the volunteers and staff who shared my vision, we had become a force. Before I had a chance to make a final decision about returning to the operating room, the chief of surgery at one of my hospitals called. "Ala, right now the city of Philadelphia needs you more than we do at the hospital. I wish you godspeed and good luck. And when you're ready to come back to the OR, we'll be here."

I wept. I was so filled with gratitude and exhaustion that all I could say was, "Thank you."

I thought about how, as an intern in Brooklyn, I had learned the lesson, *You'd better be in the hospital or be* IN *the hospital.* There was never a good excuse not to be at your post, ready and able to perform the next surgery. But now there was a very good reason, the best reason, I couldn't be in the hospital. We were doing health care the way it needed to be done in the moment.

These experiences—testing, vaccinating, watching the wheels of policymaking turn, often badly or painfully slowly—helped bring my own background into sharper relief. I had come a long way and earned the affluence and comfort that came from my efforts training to be and then practicing as a surgeon. But I was also a Philly girl with some knowledge and power now, with hustle and street cred, and a passion for the people. One who was sick and tired of being sick and tired. Tired of being told "No" or "Be patient," tired of waiting for someone to save us, someone or ones with no sense of urgency. Every experience in my life had prepared me for this crisis. I was exactly where I was supposed to be.

21

OUR OWN

An idea I'd been thinking about for months was coming into greater focus: a clinic that offered great health care right in the neighborhood, in neighborhoods like the one I had grown up in and that BDCC was serving. A one-stop shop, a more holistic approach to medicine. Behavioral health and social services. A community health center run primarily by Black Americans for Black Americans. We would turn no one away. The uninsured would be provided with a counselor to help figure out what insurance they might be eligible for, or maybe we would offer our services on a sliding fee scale. We would serve walk-ins, not just by appointment. It would be an opportunity to treat people who hadn't seen a doctor in years. To get them into programs they may not have known they were eligible for. Preventive care would be a huge priority. My goal was to create a health care center unlike anything that Kamau and I had experienced when we were growing up. I was born at Einstein Hospital, on public assistance, food stamps, often taking two or three buses to get anywhere far. I was no different from the kids and adults we were now testing and vaccinating.

Back when the idea started percolating, in summer 2020, I found myself sitting on a curb in the park with Shelah, a stellar nurse and good friend. Until then, I hadn't spoken out loud about my dream clinic, but with Shelah I did, because I thought it had to feel real if it ever was going to *be* real. I took out paper and pen and sketched out what a community health equity center somewhere in North Philly could look like. How it should function. I listed every facet of care it might offer, within financial reason.

Because of my responsibilities running BDCC, I couldn't find the time to develop the idea. But by April 2021 I knew I had to move. For weeks I scoured spaces without luck until one day we got our break: Pastor Glen Spaulding of Deliverance Evangelistic Church, one of the most historic Black churches in all of Philadelphia, had a space annexed to his church that had once been a nursery school. For five years those ten thousand square feet sat empty. We could put the health center there, at the corner of North 20th Street and West Lehigh Avenue. It was a low-income area known as Swampoodle, with one-third of its residents living in poverty. It had the lowest average life expectancy of any zip code in the city,[1] and its residents—90 percent of them Black— had suffered some of the highest infection rates. It was across the street from a high school, near public housing, right on a bus route. It was perfect.

"Okay, God," I said to Pastor Spaulding but looking up, "this looks like the plan."

Like so many people, I had to stop watching. I couldn't bear anymore to see that image of the man's knee on the other man's neck. I knew from 9/11 that I could not watch certain images. The scenes of terrified people running away from the World Trade Center, that haunting photograph of the falling man frozen in midair. You look for a moment, your mouth open, beyond horrified, and then you just can't look anymore. As a surgeon, I'm hardly squeamish. But this was something else—desperation and anguish in their purest forms.

The George Floyd video was like that: When it happened, I

watched only a few moments, then I turned my face from the screen each time. Then I realized I needed to mute it because of his cries. The revulsion became too much, and it was true again now, almost a year later, as the nation awaited the verdict in the trial of Derek Chauvin, the Minneapolis policeman, he of the infamous knee. They kept replaying the original video all over TV and the internet. You had to make an active effort to avoid it. I couldn't afford to have those images revisit my mind.

I was at the Dell Music Center doing a walkthrough in preparation for a vaccination event when the news dropped that a verdict had been reached.

Driving home, all the shops and businesses had boarded their windows in anticipation of violent protest. My husband and my brother kept checking in to make sure I made it home. The city felt like a ghost town. In my living room, I sat in front of the TV with my three sons. We held hands except for Ellison, my oldest, thirteen at the time, who stood apart and said, "I don't know why you're watching this. He's not going to jail, is he? They never do."

How do you respond to that?

As the moment approached, I was certain, like Ellison, that we would be disappointed. For all my hope about individuals, my can-do attitude, my ever-present smile, being disappointed in government action or inaction was the default for me and those in my community. Our refrain was, *It's just the way life is.* Maybe the one difference now, a positive and meaningful one, is that Black people are increasingly open about our feelings and fears, about how terrible wrongs impact us, about how vulnerable we can feel.

I expected to hear the words "Not Guilty." The verdict was read.

I sat there on the couch like that Eagles fan who can't believe her team actually won the Super Bowl.

Second-degree murder. Third-degree murder. Second-degree manslaughter.

Guilty on all three charges.

My twins and I were still holding hands, then Langston said, "Mommy, are you okay?"

"I'm okay, baby," I managed. I just lay on the couch and cried.

After the verdict, no Black person could possibly feel, *Okay, now we're good. That's never going to happen again. And if it does, the perpetrators will be found guilty.*

But I *did* think that maybe police officers, regardless of their skin color, would think a little bit more about how they approached and interacted with suspects. Maybe some police officers would start acting in a different way. They might be doing it for reasons of self-interest rather than humanity because they realized a guilty verdict was genuinely possible. But if that's what it took for change to happen, so be it. Officers no longer had a "get out of jail free" card. They could be prosecuted for their actions. Maybe they would take a moment to think about that and change their course of action.

At the end of April 2021, right before President Joe Biden's hundredth day in office, Dr. Rachel Levine, the U.S. assistant secretary of health, and her staff visited Black Doctors COVID-19 Consortium, as we vaccinated people on the grounds of Temple University. We showed Dr. (now Admiral) Levine what we were doing, then followed up afterward with a call and a debrief. I was told by her staff that I should apply for funds that Congress had earmarked for Covid relief. They made us feel we were ideal recipients, but I refused to get my hopes up. There was a painful sense of déjà vu. I had seen enormous amounts of public money funneled to the wrong people, including those who had failed spectacularly at the job. I wasn't convinced that decisions were being made in the smartest manner, with intelligent oversight. Only $600 million of the $1.9 *trillion* federal Covid-19 relief package—the CARES Act—was going to my city, the sixth-largest in America, to mitigate the virus, and I knew lots of organizations and individuals would surely pad their pockets with some of the money. The U.S. Surgeon General's office had urged community-based health organizations like BDCC in cities across the country to communicate with each other and exchange best practices, and maybe there could be a think tank? Maybe there would be money in that? And I thought: *Is that really the level of help being offered?* Millions of dollars had already been spent, much of it wastefully, on hospitals that were doing far too little for underserved communities. To give one example, the numbers coming out of one of the biggest medical centers in the city floored me: More than 80 percent of its income came from Medicare, a federal program, yet for all the people they vaccinated, what percentage were people of color? Less than 20 percent. How was that allowable?

Byron called it "show and tell." Federal funds come in, then go to the usual suspects. An influx from the CARES Act and follow-on legislation meant that there was lots of activity at first. Everyone shows up, running multiple pop-up testing and vaxxing clinics per week. The number of Covid cases start dropping. Photos are taken; stories are published in hospital newsletters. Then, the money pocketed, there's a shift down to a couple clinics a week. Then to appointment only. Then closed after one hour. Then closed altogether, as quickly as it started, the service gone, even though many more people still need it. A sham or a scam, you pick. Or, as Byron put it, show and tell: Deposit funds (Show). Announce how great you are (Tell). Soon enough, everyone moves on.

Hospitals didn't exactly bathe themselves in glory. Some were getting wheelbarrows of federal funds and *not* using it on the communities where they served. Like any corporation (and many hospitals are part of corporations), their bottom line came first. I had long been affiliated with hospitals; hospitals are necessary in the health care ecosystem; there are good and noble people who work in and run hospitals. But what went on during the pandemic lowered my already low opinion of how they often functioned and assessed priorities. The not-unheard-of profit-first, compassion-second mentality helped to explain why so many Black hospital employees didn't take the vaccine from their own institutions. (The percentage in the first two months was less than

10 percent.)[2] Early in the pandemic, many Black hospital workers felt as if they were sent constantly to work in the Covid ward, often without access to N95s or other proper PPE. So when the very same hospitals announced, "We have a vaccine for you!" you could hardly blame employees for feeling something less than trust. *Why would I put this in my body on your say-so when throughout this ordeal you have consistently left me vulnerable?* To top it off, some hospitals reportedly didn't care that their employees had Covid. Was their sickness bad enough to keep them from being on the job? No? Then stop complaining.

Bottom line.

For all my issues with city government, I had to admit that they often had limited control; the money often funneled from the federal government to the state and then to the hospitals, sometimes to the city and then the hospitals. I'm sure the city kept something for itself; everybody who could, did.

Meanwhile, as we continued vaxxing and testing, we were seeing folks who hadn't seen a doctor in a decade. We were just putting Band-Aids, often literally, on the much bigger problem of health inequity.

FEMA came through.

I knew the feds had been impressed with us, but I made sure not to expect anything from anyone. And then they delivered. It probably didn't hurt that I had posted a video on Twitter, addressed to the White House Covid response team, asking, "Where are you?"

And so BDCC finally got serious recognition for our efforts, something much more exciting and tangible than my appearance on morning TV shows: a glistening FEMA van, our new mobile unit. So comfortable. Big leather chairs with tables in the back. A freezer, a backup generator, another freezer. A restroom. We were supplied with ten tin tables, enough for five stations. Thirty folding chairs. Fifty-four cones. We could vaccinate ten people on the van at once, while hundreds could be tested outside with all the gear we now had.

Let's go!

•   •   •

Health care need not be talked about or delivered in an environment of dread. I have always wanted health care to be about joy. To heal is not just to remove what is diseased, but to get to a place of health, comfort, gratitude, grace. We cohosted a day in Strawberry Mansion, near Fairmount Park, in North Philly. We brought a DJ. We were set up in an amphitheater, cosponsored by two local radio stations, with the fire department and local police precinct helping out. Uber donated free rides to the site. We vaccinated five hundred people that day, including 490 first-time shots. Ninety-six percent of them went into the arms of African Americans. The music was fine, the mood positive. The place rocked.

Sometime in June 2021, I was told I was being considered for the position of city health commissioner, a great honor. I didn't know what exactly the role would entail—revamp all the city's clinics? Build more of them? Make sure hospitals took on a bigger responsibility in the communities they should have been serving, because they had badly missed the mark?

I didn't know if I would even want the position if it were offered. Ever since Pastor Spaulding had shown me the abandoned nursery school behind his church, my team and I were looking to do health care a new way, to do more than just be better than what had been done in the Black community in Philadelphia. Frankly, that bar was pretty low. We wanted the communities that had been systematically underserved for so long to finally do as well as everyone else. To receive health care as good, as regular, as empathetic, as well-resourced as everyone else's. Nothing less than true equity was acceptable. What we planned next would embody that idea and, I hoped, be a model for communities of color and the underserved all over the country.

22

THE POWER OF
STAYING POWER

In so many Black neighborhoods, you find lots of Chinese takeout, check-cashing places, liquor stores, salons, barbershops, and lots and lots of churches. What you *don't* find much of is vibrant health care venues. Medical offices and the like. Ambulatory care centers.

Not long ago I saw a commercial for health care set in New York City. Its tagline was "Expert care in your neighborhood." A woman exits her apartment and walks not very far to a sparkling, impressive health care edifice. Right in the neighborhood!

Every neighborhood deserves that.

Toward the end of the summer of 2021 and into the fall, as our testing and vaccination work continued, accolades for our accomplishments accumulated, and my media appearances multiplied, I looked beyond Covid. We at BDCC had broken through walls, as I myself had done time and again in my own life, and now that I had gotten to the other side of those walls, I realized I could not leave my organization behind. I could not go back to my former professional life as "just" a surgeon without trying to make some permanent difference beyond the pandemic. Once the most acute phase of the crisis passed, it would be too easy for the lessons learned to be mothballed until the next crisis; I foresaw all too clearly how our city and country could once again be reactive rather than proactive and preventive. America had broken faith with its African American population in many ways, but in the way that concerned me most directly—health and health care—I hoped to do something to repair that break.

The community deserved to feel comfortable with its local health care providers, of course. But they had to trust that the place where those people worked was not some here-today, gone-tomorrow operation. They needed a long-term investment in the neighborhood, in their individual health history, in their family's health history, so that they could trust the guidance and services they received. A huge part of our effectiveness at BDCC was our consistent presence. Community members came to trust that we weren't going away anytime soon.

To be clear, there *are* clinics in predominantly Black neighborhoods. Many of them are called commercial health agencies and FQHCs—Federally Qualified Health Centers. These clinics try to do good work. They often *do* good work. But just as often, they are not really *of* the community. That is, they're not an organic outgrowth of the community's history, values, and deepest needs. They're plunked down in neighborhoods by outsiders who don't know the people or the specific area. Sometimes those working at the FQHCs are of the community, but they are not typically the people in power. Furthermore, few of these places provide a complete range of services. This means that patients often have to scramble all over the city to receive different types of care, like testing (X-rays, MRIs, CT scans, bloodwork, etc.), pediatrics, geriatric care, mental health counseling, dentistry, eye care, legal assistance, social work, and so forth. Communities such as the one I grew up in desperately want for clinics with "wraparound services"—clinics that can meet most, or at least many, health and wellness needs all in one location, while also addressing the social determinants of health. If you're a busy working mother (is there another kind?) and your doctor writes you a prescription for a mammogram, wouldn't it be nice to get it right then and there, or at least somewhere in your neighborhood? Within walking distance? If you can't, and if it's hard for you to get all the way across town to the place that does do mammograms after working hours: that's more than just an inconvenience; that has a real effect on your health, in the short- and long-term. Multiply that by the number of people in your neighborhood and you can see how entire populations are systemically pushed into ill health and worse overall outcomes.

When BDCC first started, we soon discovered that many of the people we tested hadn't seen a doctor in years, so it was a triumph to get them to trust us. But the fact that they hadn't sought out health care of any meaningful kind in so long also meant that their well-being had been neglected and compromised in ways that had nothing to do with Covid.

One day when we were administering vaccines, I met a man in his early fifties who clearly had hypertension. Before giving him the Covid shot, I asked about his condition. He didn't get defensive; he acknowledged that I was right about his poor health. I asked what he was taking. He reached into his pocket and showed me the meds. It wasn't first-line therapy. He didn't know why it was prescribed. One thing was certain, though: It was not significantly helping his blood pressure. What he really needed was some dedicated attention: a doctor with whom he could share his background, who could order him some tests. But I had a line of people winding around the block waiting to be vaccinated. I wanted him to come back another time—But where? To see whom? In what setting? Would he? Even supposing he bought into my credentials and my knowledge and caring, was our twenty-second exchange really going to convince him?

Enough.

If these people, my people, trusted us to put swabs up their noses and tell them whether they needed to quarantine or keep going out in the world; if they trusted us to let us stick needles in their arms with a relatively new vaccine that was cleared for use only via FDA emergency authorization . . . if all that was true, then hadn't we established enough trust that they would come to us for other health needs, including routine ones?

Come fall of 2021, the dream that was housed in the annex behind Deliverance Evangelistic Church, on North 20th Street and West Lehigh Avenue, was almost complete.

The construction and renovation were funded primarily by me: I had been submitting claims to insurers and the federal government and finally started receiving reimbursements for some of the work we did at Black Doctors. I reinvested that revenue into the community, to build the center. (Some of the money I laid out would never be paid back, like what I spent to rent the first van and buy other supporting equipment needed in those initial months.) Then I also—finally!—received some government money for the health center. Not that it was dispensed quickly; this was government, after all. We were not a line item in anyone's budget.

I communicated with all seventeen members of the City Council, trying to persuade them to give our health center at minimum a five-year contract, if not a "legacy" contract, which would keep us funded so long as a need for our services existed. I sent each member a letter. I spoke with each by phone. I emailed the mayor, copying each of the seventeen council members.

But I wasn't about to wait for a definitive answer or an actual check in the mail. We forged ahead on the health center using donations and my savings. The space we had leased required massive renovation, scheduled to take six to eight months. I met with architectural engineers, medical architectural engineers, construction people. I brought my landscaper from the suburbs and told him, "People need to see life. We need trees and grass." We put in grass, even though nothing green grows in North Philadelphia. People who live in urban areas like North Philly deserve to see and smell and enjoy a little nature when they come in for medical care, just like other people do.

The center was built with love.

What we created was the result of my own vision, the input of our curator, Dori Desautel Broudy, and the incredible efforts of all the volunteers and employees, who gave so much to every detail. We were extra careful to have a sleekly paved walkway in front of the center's entrance (dug up, fixed, and smoothed so that no senior might trip over a crack; I found a paver at the eleventh hour after the first crew no-showed). We put vibrant art inside and outside the center. Each door featured a classic Philadelphia scene or figure, such as favorite daughter Marian Anderson, the legendary opera singer, and the City Hall statue of voting rights activist Octavius Catto. Patients with appointments and walk-ins alike would be greeted in the reception area by friendly, helpful staff, then led to our Welcome Center, a more inviting waiting area. We had a children's play area. We had Claims, Intake, and Social Services, the last of these situated toward the back, so that those without insurance could have private conversations. Each of the eight exam rooms was equipped with a consultation space. There were tall plants and a fish tank in the front; environments that are sensorily appealing have a beneficial effect on patient mood—particularly important in and around the mental health wing, which had three more exam rooms (or "private behavioral health spaces") and another waiting room. I chose the paint colors, the furniture, even the blood pressure cuffs and scales. Everything was designed with intention.

Services would include pediatric and adult care, blood pressure and vision screening, behavioral health, vaccinating and testing, physical examinations, phlebotomy, EKGs, preventive medicine, and education.

I officially changed our organization's name from Black Doctors COVID-19 Consortium to Black Doctors Consortium. When I first came up with the title, I anticipated the need to drop the "Covid-19" once we were focused on serving a more permanent purpose. Yet the name remained similar enough that all those people who had relied on BDCC when the pandemic was at its most intense would know it was still us—only this time we were providing access to exceptional general health care.

Contrary to what is true in so many Black neighborhoods, there actually *was* a concentration of health care venues within walking distance of our building. There were two health centers within two blocks—which, rather than have me rethink my frustration with the resources in such neighborhoods, only fueled it. Because . . . where had they been all this time? Why hadn't *they* done what it took to build trust? When we at BDCC had come to test and later vaccinate in *that exact spot* months before, we had a line of people around the block. Why were they all coming to us? Why weren't those health centers also vaccinating? The Philadelphia College of Osteopathic Medicine, with a dialysis center, was also within walking distance. So was a senior health care center in the plaza across the street from Deliverance. And there was an FQHC literally two blocks away. Why had those places—with nurses and doctors and access to certification for testing and vaccination—failed, in my eyes, to step up in the deepest, harshest days of the pandemic?

I believe the health centers were limited by bureaucracy. They wouldn't change their "business as usual" approach unless ordered to do so. But the pandemic required a decidedly *not* "business as usual" response! Administrators were desperately waiting for money so they could do extra, do the extraordinary. But the virus wasn't waiting.

We at BDCC had trust going for us. That was our not-so-secret secret.

On October 27, 2021, not even a year since I'd first envisioned it, on a clear, sunny Wednesday in the forties, the Dr. Ala Stanford Center for Health Equity (ASHE), located at 2001 W. Lehigh Avenue, and a living experiment that put the lessons I had learned to the test, had its grand opening, starting with the ribbon-cutting dedication. I decided to make the center in my name because as a Black woman doctor, I planned to be visible and vocal about what went on inside those walls.

As a bonus, maybe having my name on a beautiful building would inspire kids of all colors, but especially Black kids, especially Black *girls*,
from the neighborhood and beyond. I hoped that by letting them see
me in my white coat, see my smile, see my nice clothes, see me talking
knowledgably about important things—health—I could serve as the
kind of role model everyone needs when young. I'd like to think that
naming the center for me was less about ego and more about making—
and keeping—a promise.

After the press conference and ribbon-cutting, Pastor Spaulding led
a prayer. There were local news crews, elected officials, my parents, children, brother, husband, everyone. In the crowd, I noticed Ms. Carolyn
(MomMom) and Ellen, Will Smith's mom and sister; along with Will
and Daddio, they had been big champions of my starting something I
could truly call my own. T. J. Holmes, a reporter from *Good Morning
America*, and his camera crew had surprised me, on live television, by
unveiling a street sign showing that a portion of Lehigh Avenue had
been renamed Dr. Ala Stanford Way. Music blared and a line of honking
cars, festooned with balloons and pompoms, paraded by. My gratitude
and humility, my joy and pride and excitement, were boundless.

When I addressed those gathered, I made it clear that we were
not going anywhere. We were in the 'hood, of the 'hood. I said that
things in that community (and others I planned to expand into) could
not go back to the way they were. Health inequities and lack of access
to quality care would have to be as unacceptable for communities of
color as they are in communities that are predominately white, affluent,
and privileged. Afterward, when speaking to reporters, I got emotional
describing our hopes and expectations. We were going to take care
of everyone, from newborns to great-grandmas. We wanted to save
lives, of course, but beyond that we aimed to impact entire lifetimes.
We aimed to improve equity and access to health care for generations.
When folks came out of church and Bible study and needed a doctor,
we wanted to give them a place to go, from one place of trust to another. When people living in public housing needed a place to go, they

could come to us and get expert care; we would provide the same care they would get if they took several buses to go elsewhere. Maybe better.

Preventive care was going to be a major part of what we did and who we were. It was our goal to take care of people before the appearance of cancer or other serious disease. Colon cancer, for instance, disproportionately impacts African Americans. We would do colon cancer screenings. We would review each patient's medical history. The patient would be seen by a doctor, registered nurse, or physician assistant. We also had on-staff phlebotomists. (Specialists were scheduled to come in a couple times a month.) Prostate cancer and breast cancer are also pervasive in communities of color, so we wanted to screen for them, too—to catch them early, not after they had spread. We could handle much of that at the center, but if there were outpatient needs we couldn't meet, then we would guide and refer patients. We were going to build an electronic health records database, for ease of use and also for outreach, and after a year and a half of testing and vaccinating we had already gathered 75,000 names. When we did our first breast cancer screening workshop, we would contact all the women in the system between ages thirty and sixty.

For our first medical director I chose Dr. Velma Scantlebury, the country's first Black woman transplant surgeon, whom I first met at Pitt (where people assumed I must have been her daughter, or how else could I have been admitted there?). Some of our registered nurses were members of Chi Eta Phi, the highly regarded Black nursing sorority founded at Howard University in 1932. Despite our name, we had doctors of other ethnicities. In fact, our staff was one of the most diverse groups I've ever had the pleasure of working with, in every way. But we were predominantly Black, with more nurses than doctors. Mainly, I wanted great professionals, regardless of color, who really wanted to work with us, and finding them was no problem because so many of the staff and volunteers of BDCC had long ago signed on to our common goal and mission, short- and long-term.

How would we know if we were successful? Very simple: outcomes.

If our patients were getting good care throughout their lives, then there was every reason for them to have equally good outcomes as other groups.

I withdrew my name from consideration for city health commissioner to prevent any potential conflict-of-interest concerns over being commissioner while also running the health center. I wanted to see patients. One of the very first services we provided was giving a Covid-19 vaccine to a nine-year-old girl, her first, since the FDA had only just authorized the emergency use of the vaccine for the five- to eleven-year-old age group.

And we were in business! Though we took walk-ins, we had so many community members registering for appointments weeks and months in advance, when we could block out more time for them. For the first patients we saw, we did many initial assessments of where they were medically. While they were there, did they want an EKG? Many said yes. For some, we drew blood. Had they had a cholesterol screening? Did they know their BMI? Did they know about kidney function? Proper diet? Did they have a primary doctor? Did they want one of our doctors to be that? Did they have a gynecologist? We invited these new patients back, hoping they would return for follow-up visits, in February, March, April. We let them know we had a behavioral health/ psychology component. We weren't just generalists; we had expertise in women's health, internal medicine, GI, and more. For a multitude of problems, we hoped they would think of us. We didn't have infinite resources, of course, but we were never too far from what they might need. We focused on adult medicine on Mondays, Wednesdays, and Fridays, pediatrics on Thursdays, and administrative work on Tuesdays. We were accumulating lots of great data. Our nurses were doing an incredible job, as were our physician assistants and advanced practitioners. We had a great office manager and a great nursing director. We had a great security guard.

My colleagues and I had so many encounters like this:

John comes in for a shot. His vital signs are not great. He looks like he can't wait to leave, but we ask, "Did you know you have high blood pressure?" or "Did you take your medication today?" Reluctantly, a conversation begins. "Yeah, my diet isn't good, I know it, but I'm working all the time. I don't have time to prepare meals. That's why they call it fast food."

Or: "I really need to stop smoking, I know. I need help with that. Can you help me?"

Or (with an elderly woman): "I know why my blood pressure is up." "Why?" "I don't sleep." "Why don't you sleep?" "My son was murdered." (We weren't expecting that answer.) We started her on half a dose of a sleeping pill. My colleague followed up with her on a regular basis, to find out how she was doing. Her sleep had improved—thank God.

Or: "I need to talk to somebody Black because other folks don't get me." "Okay. Someone will be in shortly to draw blood." "What's her name?" "Tori." "Tori? That doesn't sound Black." "Well, she is." (Suspicious look from him.) "This is why I don't go to doctors. Most people don't get me." "We got you. I promise."

Or: "Can you see my husband? He hasn't been to a doctor in ten years."

We understood that every person was different, and that each was deserving of dignified, personalized treatment. That's one of the things, maybe the biggest, that's been missing in American health care for a long time—not just in Black and brown communities, not just in rural and working-class white communities, but everywhere. At ASHE, we were rectifying that. One patient at a time, one family at a time.

We were flying high. There was so much work to do but we were making a real difference and getting attention. A story in *Bloomberg News* in late October reported that Philadelphia had vaccinated a higher share of Black residents than any American city with a large Black population—more than Chicago, Baltimore, Charlotte, Columbus, Milwaukee, Memphis, Washington, Detroit—and it was largely because of BDCC's efforts. At one point Black Doctors had outpaced the city's public health department, hospitals, and FQHCs in vaccinating African Americans.

My name and the efforts of BDCC continued getting exposure, and in mid-December I was honored as a CNN Hero, with Dr. Anthony Fauci praising our operation. I received invitations from departments of medicine and surgery to come speak. Most such departments are predominantly white, or close to it, and I wondered, *Do they REALLY want me to talk about what the hell is happening out there?*

If some days I entertained thoughts of returning to surgery, and other days I pondered focusing on public advocacy, those fantasies evaporated as Christmas approached. The Omicron variant of the coronavirus, first detected in South Africa in November, had exploded around the world. Everyone was getting sick again. There were zip codes with astonishing infection rates—45 percent positive. Government offices closed. The world was shutting down again. It was PTSD for so many of us—regular people and health care providers alike—thinking back to the darkest days at the start of the pandemic in March of 2020. Two days before Christmas, a snaking line of hundreds and hundreds of people stood in the rain, wrapped around the block of the health center, waiting to get tested and vaccinated.

Our preventive care efforts were mostly put on hold. We were responding to the immediate threat, once again back to being reactive.

23

THE KIDS

Back in April 2021, before young kids were even approved for shots, I had written a proposal about vaccinating children twelve and under. It would be better, I thought, to have a plan in place when the time came than to be caught flat-footed. I outlined how I would vaccinate in schools.

In his correspondence, the health commissioner informed me that the vaccine was not yet approved for children.

Um . . . no kidding. I had acknowledged that exact fact at the beginning of my proposal. Good to see how careful the authorities read helpful documents.

The following month, May 2021, the Covid-19 vaccine was approved for emergency use for those aged twelve to fifteen. By summer, a third of twelve- to seventeen-year-olds nationally were fully vaccinated; another 10 percent had received a first dose.[1] Now, with the spread of the Omicron variant in January 2022, we were back in a full-blown public health crisis mode—and when you have such a crisis, you go to the people. Kids were back in school so that's where we went.

We started our young people's vaccination outreach at high schools, because older children—in Philadelphia, it's eleven years old and above—don't require parental consent for administration of vaccinations.

People who learn about this rule are invariably surprised. No parental consent needed for kids as young as eleven? But the rule was established decades ago, when getting other vaccines—polio, measles, etc.—was a vital public health measure, and one largely devoid of political partisanship. The powers wanted to eliminate obstacles to mass vaccination. Then—as now—many parents or caretakers couldn't get time off, certainly not paid time off, to accompany their kids to doctors' appointments for mandatory vaccines. That was one solid reason for changing the law about parental consent. There was another fundamental reason: Parents often make decisions that are not informed— and while that's their right in private, ill-informed decisions in the midst of a public health crisis affect the larger community. Since so many children needed vaccines, turning them away because they lacked a consenting adult increased the risk of a wider outbreak of measles, mumps, polio.

The no-parental-consent rule was in place long before I was born. It was never about increased personal freedom and independence; it was a public health measure. And it was never a political issue—until Covid.

We at BDCC weren't going to grab eleven-year-olds and stick needles in their arms, like it or not. We would go to schools, explain to young kids about vaccination, the benefit, and did they understand and want to do it? There would be ample publicity (or "warning," depending on your political leaning) that we were showing up at this or that school. And my team and I weren't automatons, treating each potential patient as a number; if we were confronted with a twelve-year-old or fourteen-year-old who we thought seemed particularly "young," we would abstain from administering the shot and wait for the child to come back with his or her parent or caretaker, or a message from a parent sent through the teacher. Just because we were legally within our right to give the shot didn't mean we would always go through with it.

Our first school, appropriately (for me, anyway), was Paul Robeson High School for Human Services, in West Philly. We had massively publicized when we were going to be there—Tuesday, January 18, from 9 a.m. to 2 p.m., then Thursday, January 20, from 2 p.m. to 7 p.m.—and got there early, parked our beautiful FEMA van right near the gym entrance, and set up tables and chairs outside, our stickers, our Band-Aids. The staff marched into the gym with the vaccines.

By the end of our first five-hour session, we had vaccinated 30 percent of the high school's un-vaxxed students. One student, slightly nervous (like many of them), needed to chatter through the process, and told me that his older brother had been vaccinated after contracting Covid and felt kind of crappy after the first shot.

"Okay, that can happen," I said, as I prepared the shot. "How'd he feel when he got Covid?"

"*Really* bad," said the boy.

"You think he felt worse after the shot or after coming down with Covid?"

The boy thought about it. "Covid," he concluded.

"What you just said is what I want people to hear and understand." I patted his arm. "We're all done here."

We got into a good rhythm at schools. We prioritized those with the lowest vaccination and highest infection rates. On a typical day, we vaccinated as much as one-third to one-half of the unvaccinated student population of a given school. I often took photos afterward with newly vaxxed kids, and showed genuine love for them.

We spread the vax-for-kids message. Depending on the school—high school, middle school—we had different approaches. We might have the principal send home a message with the kids in English and Spanish, or also Russian or Mandarin or other languages, depending on the community. Then I would Zoom with interested parents, explaining our process and taking questions. Or I might host a town-hall-style meeting open to the entire student body, answer questions, then meet individually with students and parents who had more questions. I toured the schools and greeted staff. I wanted everyone to know that my team and I were personally invested in their efforts and actions. Whether in person or virtually, I assured parents and school administrators that the people giving the vaccine were licensed and credentialed, that we had EMTs, nurses, doctors, and physician assistants, and that before returning to class after getting a shot, each child would be carefully monitored for fifteen to thirty minutes.

At one school, the boys' basketball team spotted us, and we succeeded at getting most of them vaccinated. The shiny decked-out FEMA van was the draw. "Are you on Instagram?" one boy asked me.

"Yep, and make sure you tag me when you post the photo."

A moment later, he said, "Wait a minute. You got a blue check." He turned to his friends. "She got a blue check!"

One Saturday I was on with Ali Velshi of MSNBC. He asked about our efforts to get the children vaccinated. Photos of the basketball team and other students were included in the segment. I returned to the school and showed them the clip of the interview. They were so hyped to see themselves on television. I was thrilled—for them and for viewers who saw the segment; it warmed my heart that these boys were being shown doing something positive.

Not everything went smoothly. We were excited to do a session at a K–8 school one Monday, along with thirty health care workers provided by FEMA. We planned to vaccinate children inside the school, and adult community members on the FEMA bus. When we arrived, though, the principal and several staff members were waiting at the door; the principal's body language told me something was wrong. She informed me that they would be calling the parents of any child who wanted to get vaccinated, including those eleven and older.

It was deeply frustrating. We had been planning the event for some time. I had already held information sessions with the teachers and parents. We'd advertised. But the school leadership decided they would do things their way. I called the Health Department and the superintendent of schools, and both agreed we were following the rules. But making sure the principal enforced the law was another matter. She just made up her own.

I did not go off on her, though I wanted to. I told the principal I was sorry this didn't work out but I had a full staff waiting to vaccinate children and we were leaving for another school to optimize our resources.

At each school, when we vaccinated the kids, we also conversed and questioned: I wanted to understand the motivations and doubts and overall thinking of the people we encountered. At assemblies I routinely asked kids and parents to submit cards explaining why they were or were not getting vaxxed. Among the reasons in favor?

Because it's convenient.

So I can play football.

To play basketball.

So I can participate in extracurriculars.

I want a job.

Among the reasons against?

It's a hoax.

My religion doesn't allow it.

It gives you Covid.

I'm afraid of needles.

My grandfather will take my PlayStation.

None of my friends are getting it.

I was glad none of these Black teens shared a reason like, *Because of the atrocities of the past, I have no trust in the medical establishment.* None of that. For most, it was about convenience and opportunity.

Among the reasons parents gave for not getting vaccinated:

Can't get off work.

Who's gonna watch my kids if it's me getting the shot?

I don't have a doctor. I thought I needed one to get a shot.

I also got answers from parents that betrayed a fundamental distrust or feeling of helplessness:

I don't trust Biden and Harris.

Who does my employer think they are telling me I have to get this vaccine?

These reactions were all about control, or lack thereof. When there's no major aspect in your life that you have control over—not your job or your living quarters or your neighborhood or your time—then maybe the only significant control you can exert is over what you put in your body and your children's. If someone seems to be taking away that right, then you become adversarial. And that kind of reaction, whether its root is ignorance or anger or something else, can have generational effects, because the apple doesn't fall far from the tree. Once, at my son Ellison's middle school basketball game, I saw a sea of unmasked parents in the stands. It was a habit for me to carry a box of masks. Here we were, indoors, mid-pandemic. The league had already canceled games due to Covid outbreaks. I began handing out masks, smiling as I said, "Don't we want the kids to keep playing? Don't we want them to be safe?" They nodded; they didn't look resentful. Without that attitude change in parents, I felt, we were just breeding a new generation of skeptics. Kids won't wear masks if their parents won't. They follow what they see.

At one high school we visited, a seventeen-year-old told me she really wanted to get vaccinated but that every time she talked about it with her mom, the answer was no. "I can't go to restaurants with my friends. I can't go to the prom without it." We talked some more and then I said, "Well, let's get you vaccinated."

She was excited but I could see the wheels spinning. "What if one day my mom decides she wants me to get vaccinated?"

"You come find me. Bring your mom and we'll take it from there."

I consulted with a pregnant fifteen-year-old who wanted to know if the vaccine was safe. I also had to point out to her that she should be wearing a mask, for her safety and the baby's. "Everybody else should wear one," she said, "so I don't have to. Or get vaccinated. Because you guys should be protecting *me*."

We vaccinated a girl who had gotten into a U of Penn summer program and couldn't attend without it, but her African mother had lots of questions and spoke only Swahili. One of our nurses had a friend in North Carolina who spoke Swahili, so we got her on FaceTime to translate as I answered the mom's questions. The mother finally agreed. Her initial objection, as with many, was that the vaccine wasn't safe. She didn't trust it. But I went down the whole list. "I got mine more than a year ago and it didn't give me Covid. It's protected me. I'm not a zombie. I didn't get cancer. It's not a government conspiracy. I'm not being tracked."

"How do you know?"

"The only thing tracking me is my Apple watch and my phone. Not anything in my bloodstream. And it's not annihilating the Black race. If it is, that's because most of the white people have gotten it and most of us haven't, so we're getting a lot more Covid and dying a lot more from it than they are."

I said a version of that to packed school auditoriums, as well. I focused on what vaccination meant for children of color. That even if they knew someone who got sick from Covid and got better, it could be worse for them next time, or worse for someone else in their household who was unvaccinated and hadn't yet gotten Covid. I argued that they themselves might get it and be fine, but they could infect a grandparent, and that person could get very sick; the "Do it for grandma" speech works much better than the "Do it for humanity" speech. The kids were so quiet, listening to everything I said. They were beautiful. Many were truly engaged. And some, of course, were clustered, whispering or talking to each other or looking at their phones, paying no attention.

At those assemblies I played a video featuring me in my white doctor's coat talking with Will Smith about being from Philly, then a clip of Dr. Fauci talking about me, with music from the rapper Meek Mill, another hometown favorite, playing in the background. I included a clip of me on CNN. I wanted to confer legitimacy. When the video was over, I asked everyone to raise their hand if they knew someone who had been really sick with Covid, or hospitalized with it, or died from it. It was sobering to see so many hands go up, and I'm sure the kids felt that weight, too. If there were parents in the audience, I made sure to say that I wasn't telling anyone what to do with their children, that I was a mother myself and didn't want anyone telling me what to do with mine. But I also emphasized the reality. I explained that more kids were contracting these more infectious (though perhaps less deadly) variants of Covid, and that more kids were landing in the hospital, including kids of color. It was a real dance to provide facts without sounding like a doomsayer and freaking everyone out.

I loved it when a principal or teacher chimed in with support. One told me, in front of a packed auditorium, "I just got vaccinated for the first time! You inspired me." There were other particularly gratifying moments. The day I vaccinated a bunch of Ellison's track teammates, I asked the kids who wanted to go first. I was so proud when Ellison raised his hand, making it easier all around.

One teacher I met simply would not be vaccinated. She insisted on wearing a mask and getting tested several times a week. Unfortunately, she wasn't alone. For quite a few teachers who were also masking and frequently testing, the refrain was, "I'm just not ready for the vaccine." I didn't push. I just told them that if they wanted to talk about it, I'd be there. And if they changed their mind, we were around, somewhere, from Monday through Saturday.

I had quite a few parents who wanted to beat my ass, especially the ones of children ages eleven, twelve, and thirteen. "Don't you talk to my kid about vaccine," said one mother, with her twelve-year-old daughter quietly standing beside her.

"Listen, I'm just letting you know the facts," I said. "These are not my rules. These are the rules of the city of Philadelphia. And in case your child didn't know that the vaccine is available, I'm also letting her know." The children's advocate in me never left.

"Well, my kids are with me all the time. So they're not getting anything."

"I hear you. That's fine. But I'm letting them"—and here I made eye contact with the girl—"I'm letting them know, too."

24

OWNING IT

I accepted the invitations.

I talked to medical school departments of surgery and to other groups of doctors about what I'd been doing for close to two years, what hospitals were not doing, why it was necessary for me to have taken time off from being a pediatric surgeon to pursue this, *all in*. I made sure to tell some fun stories about adventures in testing and vaccination, to humanize the experience. But, doctors being doctors, I also talked statistics, vaccination rates, increases and decreases in hospitalizations and deaths. So much of what we physicians do is driven by numbers, objectivity, probability, not subjective feeling. We go by what's reproducible and evidence-based and worthy of publication, which can equal funding. That's what we live by.

There's an absurdity to that, though. Because if it really *was* all about the data, then racism and sexism in medicine would have disappeared a long time ago. Right? Because if a problem with undeniable statistical support—say, rates of infection, hospitalization, and death from a highly spreadable virus in Population B that are way higher than in Population W—then you would of course address that first, not last. There would be no subjectivity to it. There would be no question as to how to proceed. You wouldn't treat things as if statistical evidence didn't exist, or as if the evidence was the opposite of what it was, as if some people mattered more than others in some subjective sense. You would respond to the greatest objective need. Especially because when one person is healthy, we are all better for it, as is the health ecosystem, the economy, and society.

I pointed out to my audiences a harsh, obvious truth about human beings, including us doctors: When a problem doesn't impact us, or maybe people who look like us, we feel less urgency to solve it. That's a fact. Call it our unconscious bias, but people naturally have an affinity for people like themselves. We all do. There's a commonality, a culture we automatically get, a shared empathy. It permeates decision-making, resource allocation, selection. It allows us literally to look right past those in greatest need. Maybe we have moved past more conscious versions of bias—redlining was about as conscious as it gets—but whether our biases were unconscious (harder to spot, easier to address) or conscious (easier to spot, very hard to change), the results of these biases were ongoing, systemic, and tragic.

I pointed out to my audience what I thought were indisputable facts. To a large extent, the health of the individual begins with the health of their community. But so many communities are ensnared in the quiet discrimination of low expectations. What they need—what everyone needs and expects—is a place brimming with vitality and potential. What happens when that vitality gets sapped before it has a chance to flower? I quoted a recent study that found that Black people under the age of thirty-five were already at heightened risk for a heart attack or myocardial event.[1] The main cause? There's not just one. Certainly *a* reason is that Black Americans disproportionately suffer the traditional risk factors of heart disease—high blood pressure, obesity, diabetes—and at younger ages. Another reason is that "people living in predominantly Black neighborhoods are substantially less likely to receive bystander CPR than white people."[2] But I'm confident that another, broader reason is at play: stress. Too many African Americans live in tough neighborhoods, have tough lives. How do you counsel someone to reduce the stress in their life when the stress comes from where they lay their very head? And from the places where they learn, work, eat, commute, and do most activities in between? "It is cruel jest to say to a bootless man," said Dr. King, "that he ought to lift himself by his own bootstraps."

I pointed out to my audience that we *know* what the problem of health care inequity looks like. The dilapidated facilities. The overworked staffs. The pleading for basic supplies. The fragmentation of care. The last-in-line treatment. The lack of role models among caregivers, especially those with the most authority. And, of course, the higher rate of negative health outcomes, including shorter life expectancy, which is tied to less access, lower income, greater bias.

The mystery is not in what's wrong. It's in our failure to do enough to address these inequities. How could we, as medical professionals, make a difference? In the short term and long term? For the aged and the newborns and everyone in between?

I'd like to believe my talks had some impact and made some of my colleagues examine what it really means to be a provider of care. When you are trained in medicine, you're taught to assess objectively the patient's problem and figure out the best way to improve their situation. In this case, if the "patient" is "health care for Black America," and we assess the problem objectively, then we must conclude not only that there *is* a very real problem, one that persists to this day, but that we have a responsibility—as doctors, as Americans, as human beings—to face it head-on and do something about it. If we look the other way, then we're culpable. At many of my talks I closed by asking my audience to go home and look in the mirror and ask themselves: How am I contributing to the health disparities that persist in this country?

When I was done, there was silence. They had nothing to say. I hoped that meant they were pondering how they could be part of the solution.

I always wanted to be the healer. As much as I loved and continue to love pediatric surgery, as hard as I worked to become one of the select few who achieve the honor to do that, I discovered how much I loved primary care, too. I think I could have been pretty happy doing house calls, in North Philly, following my time in medical school and residency. (And because primary care requires fewer years of training, I would have been out in the world doing it way sooner, before I was thirty!) I would have loved taking care of my people like that. But primary care did not have the prestige of other specialties. It didn't get the same respect. It didn't pay nearly as well. It wasn't as intense and engaging as surgery, and I was wired for that.

Now, in the prime of my professional life, I had found exactly what I needed to be doing. I thought of how my pastor, Reverend Mitchell, had once asked me about starting a hospital in Haiti, and the first thought that came to me: *Great idea . . . but wow that sounds really hard.*

My next thought, *There's a lot of work to do at home.*

Opening the clinic was a great first step but only a step. I imagined clinics like it all over the place. I hoped the center could be a model not only for Philadelphia but for the country, showing doctors and medical practitioners in all fifty states how to start addressing health care disparities for communities of color and overlooked rural communities. What would make that happen?

One of the major problems with health care is the quality and experience of the provider—that is, Who is providing your care? Is it someone empathetic to you? Someone who knows your struggle? For these clinics to work well, we would need to find and train health care leaders in diverse communities who were culturally competent and culturally appropriate—that is, leaders who understood that their own beliefs and values may differ from others, and who supported young people upholding their own identities. It would require cultural humility. As leaders, they would need to understand the lived experiences of those they wished to help. They would need to ensure that the care they provided was equitable, and that their patients knew, explicitly, that they were being treated with the same standard as everyone else, yet the care was unique to them as individuals. We would need leaders who take real action, and don't take no for an answer.

That's how trust is born and sustained. Without it, trust dies.

We began looking to expand beyond the North Philly location. We had our eyes on another facility, on Germantown Avenue, close to an elementary school. That was going to be our trademark: Plant ourselves right in the community, where we could easily reach people and touch their lives. Was it difficult to imagine such expansion? Not really. 1 Corinthians 2:9: "Eye hath not seen, nor ear heard, neither have entered into the heart of man, the things which God hath prepared for them that love Him." Until you make something happen, it may seem impossible. I had faced obstacles in my life, but lack of belief was never really one of them. My faith was always driving me. I believed we had been brought this far for a reason.

Long after I'm old and gone, I want the Center for Health Equity still to be there, providing care, extending and saving lives.

25

THE SOCIAL DETERMINANTS OF HEALTH

In the first months of 2022, my increasingly public profile meant lots of phone calls, texts, and emails from people in high places. More invitations to speak, including offers to deliver the commencement address at several of my alma maters, among them Penn State-Behrend, Penn State University Park, Penn State College of Medicine, and the University of Pittsburgh Medical Center. (If a fortune-teller had told me during my darkest days at each of those institutions that one day I would be asked to deliver their commencement address, I would have thought she was high. And asked for a refund.) I was invited to give a TEDx Talk at the University of Pennsylvania, which thrilled me. There were headhunting inquiries and job interviews. Nonprofits, corporations, academia. I was intrigued by a new challenge, while working at a job I loved and that fulfilled me—overseeing my health center. But why not see what these other organizations might enable me to do? Some seemed well-intentioned but lacked a coherent vision. Some lacked the resources to do what they said they wanted to. I needed to figure out which, if any, would allow me to have the most impact. A couple of organizations recruited me, interviewed me more than once, then turned me down, and I couldn't help but think: *Hey, YOU called ME! Remember?* I really hoped I hadn't made their list just so they could check the "diversity/equity in hiring (or at least interviewing)" box.

Then the White House came calling. The White House!

After many rounds of interviews—many, many—and lots of background checks, I was offered the position of regional director of the United States Department of Health and Human Services. HHS divides the U.S. into ten regions, and mine would be Region 3, the mighty Mid-Atlantic, which includes Pennsylvania, Virginia, West Virginia, Maryland, Delaware, and the District of Columbia, a particularly diverse stretch of the country. The office was based in Philadelphia.

The regional director works with divisions of various federal health care agencies, including (to name a few) the Centers for Medicare and Medicaid Services (CMS), the Health Resources and Services Administration (HRSA), the Administration for Children and Families (ACF), and the Substance Abuse and Mental Health Services Administration (SAMHSA). The budget was in the billions of dollars. HHS's mission was massive: "to enhance the health and well-being of all Americans, by providing for effective health and human services and by fostering sound, sustained advances in the sciences underlying medicine, public health, and social services."

I knew the Philadelphia Department of Health mission statement by heart and had been disappointed by their failure to live up to their credo during the pandemic. I didn't want to start out cynical about what another government agency—a way bigger one—was promising.

In April of 2022, after much consideration, I said yes to the HHS job . . . Yes!

In two years I had gone from squeezing colleagues for unused test kits and PPE to advising on best health practices for the entire nation, appointed by the president of the United States.

Not bad for a girl from North Philly.

•   •   •

Being in the public sector I got a look at health care from a very different perspective. I talked to governors, mayors, tribal leaders, partners, and citizens throughout the region and beyond. For Americans in my region, I was the "front door" to the HHS. My incredible staff kept me from getting overwhelmed by all that lay in front of us: continuing Covid-19 vaccination and treatment; expanding access to health care, especially for marginalized communities; implementing a new strategy for drug overdose prevention; lowering the cost of hearing aids by making them available over-the-counter; elevating mental health resources and visibility, which the Biden administration had made a priority, including the rollout of a new mental health and suicide hotline (#988); bringing down prescription drug costs; addressing monkeypox; reducing infant mortality and improving maternal health; strengthening home health care; and lowering the cost of care generally, not to mention my daily interactions with citizens who had questions about so many aspects of health care . . . yeah, we were busy.

I had the privilege of great power and wasn't about to squander it. One of my goals was to make the conversation about persistent racial inequities in health care *real*, not just a talking point or two. To sharpen the message, it needed to be simplified, which wasn't hard.

The social determinants of health.

That phrase tells the whole story. It's at the heart of health disparities.

Health care doesn't occur solely in the hospital, the clinic, the physician's office. It happens in the community. If a community is to live in better health, then the social determinants of health must be understood and addressed. What are the forces that encumber people from living in good health, in better health? What does a community need to flourish?

A community must have, at minimum, four elements to thrive:

- Food—groceries, supermarkets, access to healthy food
- Education—schools with resources, other places to learn

- Money—banks, financial institutions
- Health care—ambulatory care centers, hospitals, medical personnel

Let's look more deeply at each.

Food

As a doctor, I know it's imperative for us to improve the nutrition level in the diet of so many young Black people. Eating processed foods high in carbohydrates, sugar, and salt significantly increases the risk of obesity, type 2 diabetes, heart disease, and so many other terrible health outcomes, and at surprisingly young ages. Yet so many people will blame Black people for their food choices. Unfortunately, the offerings in many poor, predominantly Black neighborhoods make it very difficult for even the most well-meaning parents to keep kids from eating crap and drinking soda and sugary juice. Some of these neighborhoods are "food deserts": communities with few conveniently situated places that offer whole, fresh foods, including vegetables, that provide proper nutrients. And these food deserts don't exist by accident: One principle of redlining was to disincentivize developers from building businesses—including grocery stores—in Black communities. Banks would not lend to "risky" businesses in redlined zip codes, or they would offer to do so only at such astronomical interest rates that it widely discouraged development. Hence, even today, there are often no good grocery stores within walking distance. (A McDonald's sits across the street from my health center. What does that say?) Many people in these same communities don't have cars, so if the shopping is beyond walking range, then they're taking the bus.

That was me growing up: Kamau and I took public transportation everywhere. When we went to the grocery store, part of the reason we didn't buy lots of food was because we didn't have much money. But even if we did, we'd still have had to lug it all home, which meant putting it in the broken shopping cart, hoping the wheel didn't fall off this time, yanking it up the three steps to get on the bus, then maneuvering it down the center aisle. So "choice" was compromised. The fruits and vegetables we got in the stores closer to us weren't as fresh, if they were even in stock. And those neighborhood groceries were not exactly safe. So we ended up, like so many people in our circumstances, buying prepared food cooked with lots of salt and lots of sugar. I applaud Michelle Obama's Let's Move! campaign to reduce childhood obesity by promoting healthy eating and exercise, but without real follow-up, without actual affordable, well-stocked grocery stores in your neighborhood, I don't know that it can have much of a lasting positive impact.

Suppose Black neighborhoods offered easier access to nutritious, unprocessed food; suppose more Black adults had the financial means to have time at home to prepare meals. How much better would Black health be then? Along with your genetic makeup, nothing likely impacts your health more than the food you put in your body. With such a poor diet starting at such a young age, far too many Black children miss developmental milestones; so do other poor children of color, and poor white children. Their opportunities down the road will suffer. In a way, it's a form of dietary redlining.

Education

What is the state of early childhood education in the community? Of vocational training? Of higher education?

The schools in predominantly Black neighborhoods are not resourced as well as schools in white neighborhoods. The Commonwealth of Pennsylvania spends far more money per student in affluent neighborhoods than poor ones.[1] Other funds to support schools come from real estate taxes from homeownership, which is dramatically lower in poor Black neighborhoods, where most rent and live in HUD/public housing: That's how Black communities were *intentionally designed*.

Almost three in four Black children attend a high-poverty school (more than half the kids are eligible for free or reduced-price lunch); fewer than one in three white children do.[2] Black students are more likely to be in schools with novice, less qualified, or less well-paid teachers. This widespread disparity has been happening for generations. How does that impact a community, a race of people?

In 2020, the rate of college or graduate school enrollment for Black males eighteen to twenty-four was 31 percent; for Black females it was 40 percent.[3] But in the decade from 2010 to 2020, Black college enrollment had plummeted by more than 10 percent[4]. (Among Hispanic students over the same time period, enrollment increased by almost 50 percent, and it also increased, though at a much lower rate, among Asian Americans.) That downturn sped up at the end of the decade into the new one: Black student enrollment fell 18 percent from fall 2019 to fall 2021, and the decline was steeper for men.[5] Best-Colleges.com noted in 2022 that "colleges are experiencing a Black male enrollment crisis nationwide."[6] There are multiple reasons for this, including that Black youths are more likely than their non-Black counterparts to be suspended in secondary school and that Black male students lack access to role models in education.[7] On *PBS NewsHour*, Christopher Emdin of Columbia Teachers College said that "50 percent of public-school students [are] of color. . . . Eighty-two percent of those teachers are . . . white. Less than 2 percent of those who teach are black males."[8]

Just under 10 percent of all K–12 school principals are Black; almost 80 percent are non-Hispanic white.[9] We don't have enough providers that look like the people we serve. And students don't have enough teachers that look like them or understand them culturally. That also contributes to high rates of detention and suspension.

As I've written, patients of color do better with doctors of color.[10] So we need more concerted development in the health professions. Earlier in the book I cited the disturbingly low numbers of Black men and women in some medical professions, and how the percentages are even lower for surgeons. But how could anyone expect those numbers to be higher when the pipeline *into* medical school is so small?

Not everybody wants to be a doctor. Not everyone has the grades, test scores, passion, ambition, and persistence to do it. But if there are so few role models at the start who might inspire Black youth to go into medical fields, and the local health care environment is poorly resourced rather than nurturing, then why would the number of doctors increase significantly? How can we expect there to be a robust number pursuing other professional degrees, in law, engineering, education, architecture, etc.? It's pure math: If the original number is so small, *of course* there will be so few Black doctors and other professionals! What you put in is what you get out.

It all starts way back. We all know this. We all lament this. We need to carve a path and instill hope at the elementary school level, or even before, if we're going to pump up those numbers. After all, I started dreaming about being a doctor when I was eight!

We are breaking a promise to children if we tell them they can be anything they want and then don't make it possible for them to do so. The barriers I faced, and that so many other minority medical students face, must be demolished. Black doctors must take their place on academic boards and committees. More Black doctors should be attendings, interns, residents, and fellows. But the attrition rate in medical school for Black students is alarmingly high.[11] Medical school should be as close to free as possible (some of them are). Medical student debt can crush a dream. Many students wind up owing more than $300,000, so they're forced to choose higher-paying jobs and specialties that take them away from poor and working-class communities, so they can pay off their loans.[12]

Money

Many people would like to believe that poverty is the fault of the impoverished. Is it? Far too often it's the result of a history of inequity and inaccessibility and tipped scales, ingrained over generations. The effect of redlining wasn't a ripple; it was a tsunami. Economic stress, particularly when it's the result of entrenched policy, affects the current generation and the generation coming up. It has the gall to affect the next generation after that, the one in the wombs of mothers, as stress hormones shape a baby's brain.

Lack of wealth may be felt in various ways: fewer good jobs (because of the lack of good education, lack of proximity, lack of generational sharing of information and connections—see my experience as a premed and in medical school). It may also be felt in the lack of investment in the neighborhoods where so many Black people grow up. Again, this was the very point of redlining: to create maps in which predominantly Black neighborhoods were colored red, signaling a risky investment for those with money. Risky places for building homes, businesses, schools, hospitals. It becomes a vicious circle. Without capital flowing into these communities, with their largely Black and brown population, there's no real transformational development happening. If no real development is happening, then investors remain wary about putting in their money. It's too big a risk.

That's why I put my health care center in one of the poorest zip codes in Philadelphia.

So many of these communities have incredible potential. People with vision can actually see a future of economic vibrancy. Unfortunately, for many developers that means a future in which gentrification has pushed current residents out. That can't be the only way. How do we invest in and improve these neighborhoods without transforming them into largely affluent white enclaves, and where the population of color has been forced to migrate to another neglected part of town? I won't presume to attempt an answer here to such a profound question. But that's one of the challenges that needs to be solved satisfactorily *for the people with roots in these neighborhoods*. As the saying goes: The only real estate is real estate. You can't build more land. What's there is what's there, so the land in these communities becomes valuable, at some point. Too often, though, that point is not while the people who've lived there for so long inhabit it.

Money affects everything—the quality of housing, mass transportation, safety, a neighborhood's parks and playgrounds or lack thereof. When people suffer from deep, constant economic stress, without the safety net of generational wealth or the pride and opportunity that come with robust investment in their communities and themselves, of *course* it will have a massive effect on their health, and not in a good way.

Health Care

Achieving health equity and health care equity are complex. There are so many factors, including the three we've just discussed. It's estimated that when an emergency warrants your visiting a hospital, approximately 80 percent of your ultimate success in getting out of there is determined by things that happened to you outside the hospital, with 20 percent determined by the controlled environment of the hospital and the skill of the medical staff. I disagree. I think it's closer to a 50/50 split. (With certain congenital conditions, of course, the ratio would be much different.) If poor, predominantly Black communities had regular access to higher-quality medical facilities and ambulatory care centers, like the ones that tend to exist in more affluent, white-majority communities, don't you think the former population would get more regular checkups for blood pressure, cholesterol levels, emotional wellness, and the like? Suppose in Black-majority neighborhoods the residents could make medical appointments without much hassle, and the majority of the appointments weren't reserved for patients with private insurance—how much would that improve stress level and overall health? Suppose the medical clinic they frequented actually offered all the major subspecialty services—wraparound care—and it was located in a shiny, freshly painted building, next to a parking lot where the cars were secure, or along a bus or subway route convenient to home, and suppose the people working in the clinic looked energetic and happy? What about a fitness club right in the neighborhood, offering low-cost membership? And multiple markets nearby with fresh, nutritious food? That would help, but it still doesn't address the trust factor. How much do Black Americans trust the health care system? How much should they trust it? Health care providers must acknowledge the bias they bring into the exam room, the operating room, and to every patient encounter.

Health care inequity is not all about race. Every white person who receives substandard health care, including so many of those in rural communities, deserves better, too.

We will not eradicate disparities in health and health care without eradicating inequities in the areas listed above. We simply cannot improve outcomes without addressing and changing the environment where these inequities breed and persist. The concept of "social determinants of health" has been around for a century and a half, dating back to the Jim Crow era.

Approximately a hundred years later, in 1985, Margaret Heckler, President Reagan's secretary of health and human services, came out with a landmark report on Black and minority health (as I referenced earlier) that shone a light on racial disparities in health care and health outcomes, concluding that "social determinants of health have a major impact on people's health, well-being, and quality of life." I'm so thankful that she and her team did that.

But how much has changed since then? In medical school a quarter-century ago, I—along with many students and faculty of color, and many white students and faculty, too—were having discussions about this problem, about how you can't really improve health outcomes for Black people without improving education, food security, housing, jobs, and more. Here we are, today, still having the same discussion.

When will discussion turn into real action, with real results? What are the specific initiatives we must take to improve and equalize the social determinants of health?

As regional director in the Department of HHS, I had a big job with a big title, but I was restless. After all the years dealing with children and newborns and their families under the most intense circumstances, after two years of meeting with people terrified of a global virus and providing them with tests and vaccines and hopefully some measure of comfort, I felt a powerful urge to connect again with individuals. Doctor to patient. There's nothing like it.

But I couldn't give up the bully pulpit of my position. Not yet.

Fall of 2022 I returned to State College, Pennsylvania, for homecoming at Penn State, which was especially gratifying after so much time spent quarantining. I love so many things about PSU and so many of the people I met there; I wouldn't have returned for such an event if my time there were awful.

Yet, as the song goes, *There's always something there to remind me . . .*

To remind me that no matter how well I did at a big, predominantly white institution, I was first and last a Black person: Five college friends—all Black women, all Penn State graduates, all professionally accomplished, all Alpha Kappa Alpha sorority sisters—and I headed to the weekend's football game wearing white; Penn State famously has a "White Out" game (no joke) where everyone dresses in white. It makes quite a visual. (They usually face a Big Ten rival in the White Out game, making the atmosphere electric.) The five of us women were in a white Tesla, me driving, and as we pulled up to the VIP parking lot entrance, the attendant asked, "Dropping off?" as if I was the Uber driver. I flashed the VIP parking lot pass and he let us through—but of course that wasn't the end of it.

As we disembarked after parking, a white man, apparently trying to be helpful, asked, "Are you sure you're in the right place?"

As we made our way toward the tailgating, each of us wearing lanyards around our neck with "PSU Homecoming" visible on our IDs, several excited white women ran up to us and asked if we were moms of football players and which ones?

An hour or so later, settled in the President's Suite (I was invited), someone insisted on guessing which sport I had played during my time at PSU. He thought he was complimenting me by insisting that I *had* to have received a scholarship.

I had graduated from there three decades earlier. I studied and trained for almost twenty years to develop the knowledge and skill that would allow me, among other things, to save premature infants from dying, a skill that requires discipline and schooling so rigorous, less than 0.0001 percent of the world can do it.

Always something there to remind me.

In December 2022 I was invited for grand rounds at the University of Pittsburgh and to spend time with medical school students. I was also invited to speak to the departments of surgery and of pediatrics at the Children's Hospital of Pittsburgh. They rolled out the red carpet for me. The department chair at Pitt, who had shown me support when I was there twenty years earlier, was just as welcoming now. One of the trauma doctors who had helped me through the turmoil was also still there, and I thanked him for being fair to me. I also spoke with doctors who had been residents with me in that tumultuous time, and nearly everyone acknowledged that it was harder for me than it should have been; several all but apologized for any role they may have played in the unpleasantness. For a couple of them, I wondered if they truly remembered—or denied to themselves—what jackasses they had been. Then there were the ones who were *so* not Team Ala back then, and who could see that I had lately become somewhat of a public figure.

"So . . . are you still operating?" asked one. "Doing any clinical work?"

How predictable. Surgeons validate their worth by wielding a scalpel, so my interrogator must have thought this would get to me, now that I was a bureaucrat and not (for the moment, anyway) a practicing surgeon. But their dagger could not penetrate my flesh anymore. I just smiled and thought, *Damn, y'all haven't changed a bit.*

Later, when I gave my lecture in a big auditorium, I made sure to find faces in the audience that looked like mine. I wondered how those young doctors were holding up.

And I couldn't help but think of, well, my own. My hometown. What else could I do to make an actual positive difference?

26

WE KNOW WHAT'S BROKEN. NOW LET'S FIX IT.

How can we restore the broken promise of health equity in America?

Acknowledge. Believe. Identify. Act. Share.

As an HHS regional director, I developed a presentation that I hoped would rouse people to action. I gave a version of it to numerous audiences. Now, I will share it with you.

1. ACKNOWLEDGE that health disparities exist.

It pains me that this should be one of the five points—especially in 2024—but it is. It's a cliché to say, but without recognizing the problem, there's no way to solve it. If people don't acknowledge there's a problem, then *that's* a problem.

On average, Black Americans have meaningfully worse health than white Americans. At birth, if you are Black, your life expectancy is more than a half-decade shorter than if you are white.[1] Black infants die at a rate more than double that of white infants.[2] Pregnancy-related mortality for Black women is more than three times higher than for white women.[3] And on and on. There are differences in Hispanic and Asian American health outcomes, of course, but I am focused here on Black health outcomes. The health disparities must be acknowledged, so that we can have a meaningful discussion about why and what to do about it.

To quote the title of an op-ed in *U.S. News & World Report*: "Being black is bad for your health."[4] That's the result of a foundational fact about America: It created generational wealth for one group, while another group was pressed into free or low-cost labor so the first group could maintain and grow that wealth. One group was able to transfer generational wealth, the other generational grief.

No one living created these practices. But—as simply put as I can—one group benefited and the other did not. There's no blame or shame. But once we acknowledge this, what will we do differently? Individually and collectively?

2. BELIEVE that health disparities exist because of systemic institutional practices, racist acts, and modern-day continuance of historical beliefs.

Acknowledgment is the first step, genuine belief the next.

We are in a futile, vicious cycle right now. Without addressing the enormous inequity that is determined largely by race and class, we'll continue to see Black people, other people of color, and poor people disproportionately facing diminished access and inadequate resources, resulting in worse health outcomes, including earlier death. And as long as those worse outcomes happen, the more it gives cover and license to those who believe that personal responsibility (controlled by one person and one person alone) or genetic makeup (out of one's control) is the root cause.

Remember the paper I presented at my own hospital, which showed that Hispanic children who underwent surgery for midgut volvulus had worse health outcomes than white children? *After* we had eliminated other potential factors? And my surgical colleague simply refused to believe the results? Our data must be flawed, he said. How could racism be involved? Impossible! Slanderous!

I don't at all think he was racist, or that doctors or hospital staff treated Hispanic children any less well than they did others. But in so many studies, race has been shown to be a "risk factor." Not for every individual, procedure, or medical facility, of course, but for enough to have what medical people call statistical significance.

People must believe that redlined neighborhoods around the country were *systemically* deprived of quality essential resources, or often any resources period, because of the skin color of those who lived there. In Philadelphia, the hospitals in the zips we served during Covid are almost uniformly subpar to other hospitals in the city. How could the inequality in neighborhoods *not* impact the quality of health care, and thus health outcomes, for the Black and brown people who have lived there for generations?

Life expectancy is linked to metrics like wealth, labor protections, affordable housing, education—those stubborn social determinants of health. These are not mere correlations but *causes* of health inequity, and for the longest time they have been heavily skewed based on race. The problem of racial disparities in health care is still with us. After the Covid pandemic, how can anyone believe otherwise? The inequity was once again brought into stark relief for me by a paper published in mid-2022 titled "The Relationship of Historical Redlining with Present-Day Neighborhood Environmental and Health Outcomes."[5]

One seemingly small but encouraging step was taken by St. Christopher's Hospital for Children, which serves a large Latino and Black population: In their outpatient office, a prominently placed poster reads, in summary: "We realize there are multiple factors that determine health, including social determinants like housing, education, employment, financial stability, and healthcare access and quality. If you are having a problem with any of these factors, please let your healthcare provider know." Many families of hospitalized children are dealing with more than a particular distressing medical situation— there may be aggressive landlords, no heat, food insecurity, unemployment, threats of deportation, etc., which can have a material effect on the child's recovery and long-term health. This statement goes past acknowledging the problem, and names potential root causes, while the institution provides support and action to address and help solve the problem.

As importantly, we must believe that achieving health equity benefits us all. (And, conversely, that not achieving health equity hurts us all.) According to the Kaiser Family Foundation, minority health determines the health of the nation.[6] What do they mean by that? "Addressing disparities is important not only from a social justice standpoint," reads their policy paper, "but for improving our nation's overall health and economic prosperity." Each of us in health care must think of health inequity not as someone else's problem, but as a situation that each of us can help solve for the benefit of others and ourselves.

"An ounce of prevention is worth a pound of cure" is not some silly old saying. Funding preventive care costs pennies on the dollar compared to the expense of, say, taking care of a forty-year-old diabetic who's had a stroke, multiplied by the countless individuals suffering that fate. In such a case, that person is now a far less productive member of society. Maybe he can't feed himself. Maybe she can no longer drive or support her family. Think of all the dollars—often taxpayer dollars—that go to caring for that person, in their physically diminished state, for years and years. Isn't that evidence that we are all helped by achieving health equity, and all hurt by keeping things the way they are?

If fairness, humanity, and economic and cultural vibrancy aren't motivation enough for our all working toward addressing health disparities driven by skin color, there's also this: The United States is diversifying faster than predicted, and people of color are projected to make up more than half of the American population in 2050. (In 2020, it was 39 percent.[7])

Dr. Alberto Peña, my brilliant mentor in Cincinnati, once told me, "the eyes see only what the mind suspects." He meant it about surgery: You won't be on the lookout for aberrant anatomy, for example, if you haven't read about it in a textbook or done the procedure previously. In his wisdom, though, the statement is just as true about life. Don't believe racism exists and you won't see it. We won't work toward eradicating racial inequities in the world unless and until we believe that they are, in fact, racial inequities.

We need not search for all kinds of explanations. The main reason is right in front of us.

3. IDENTIFY how you can be most impactful in eradicating disparity.

You may wonder: *What can I do?*

You don't need a big title. You don't need a big budget. You need to identify your strengths, the unique opportunities you have to improve things, your skills and talents to impact a community, and the path to get going. When you do all that, you will feel a sense of inevitability, purpose, and peace. When we were testing and vaccinating people, we knew that we were exactly where we needed to be. We knew if we were present and persistent, we would gain trust and thus make an impact. Everyone can play a role.

So . . . what can you do? What role can you play?

If your organization's role is making policy or passing legislation or providing funding, then maybe the most important point to identify is this: Is what you're currently doing working? Is it actually addressing and reducing disparity? Is it not helping at all? Could it even be exacerbating it? How would you go about answering that? (More on that in a bit. This step is about identifying.)

What can you as an individual do? Suppose you're a hairdresser in the community. You've probably gained trust over the years with your clientele of women who mostly fall in a certain age range. What can you do to have an impact?

Suppose you're a bus driver who works for SEPTA. You know you have a captive audience every day. What message to them might move the needle?

Suppose you're a single parent, working such long days that you're never able to see a doctor during normal business hours. (Your kids are fortunately able to get to the doctor, unsupervised.) How do you make sure to take better care of yourself, which translates to taking better care of your loved ones?

There are countless ways to have impact, both on your own and especially when collaborating with organizations whose mission is to eradicate health disparities.

One of my mantras as a health care provider for vulnerable groups: If I'm getting up, going to work in a hospital or medical office or operating room, then going home, I'm not doing enough. If I'm comfortable and not inconvenienced, I'm not doing enough.

The message applies to everyone. Figure out how you as an individual or your organization can help.

4. ACT in your role to eradicate disparity.

Government, community-based organizations, hospitals, philanthropies, doctors and other health care professionals, patients: Everyone must act, and acting in collaboration is likelier to have impact than acting within silos. The problem is too big and persistent for one hand not to know what the other hand is doing. The decision-makers have the power to change the culture and place emphasis on health equity. The decision to do so must come from the top.

The federal government provides the most money, at a level no one else matches. It provides guidance, such as the recent White House Executive Order on "Advancing Racial Equity and Support for Underserved Communities Through the Federal Government Cooperative."

But Barack Obama probably said it best: "Change doesn't come *from* Washington. It comes *to* Washington." One immediate, meaningful action that I'd love to see bureaucracies take, and that would have helped us at Black Doctors, is making the application process saner and more user-friendly. At times, I found it surreal and ludicrous that to get approved to vaccinate vulnerable Philadelphians in a global emergency, it took me close to twenty-four hours (no exaggeration) to fill out forms. Why the unnecessary hurdles and roadblocks?

Who else must act, and how?

Doctors must give their patients what they need. I hope most doctors already know this, but there's so much that our patients can teach us. It's cultural humility, plain and simple. How are we to know all the answers to our patients' problem without getting input from them? For many doctors, it's more or less a paradigm shift to hear and listen to patients and their families, and to create a safe space for this meaningful exchange to occur. Patients genuinely have to feel the doctor's willingness to be present, and in a judgment-free zone. This is trust-building. It's how we achieve long-term health. We must take time to discuss the importance of screening tests, and more time to explain the results. Let's work to rewrite the story, so that white doctors are spending as much time discussing medical treatment and options with Black patients as they are with white ones. It doesn't help to say "smoking is bad for you" or "you need to decrease the stress in your life and exercise more" without also providing a feasible smoking cessation program, tips for stress relief, and recommendations for accessible, safe locations to exercise.

Far too often, as I wrote earlier, there are racially related explanations for poor diet, smoking, obesity, and so forth, and they are not changed as easily as flipping a switch. We know that smoking and vaping are over-targeted to communities of color. Doctors need to focus on the behavior and then work to modify it, but also to understand the "upstream" input that caused it, not just the "downstream" result. It's up to us, all Black and white and brown doctors, to make sure that Black patients know that we are there to help make and keep them healthy, whatever it takes. Then it's up to them to follow through, with our support. We are *partners* in preventive maintenance of their health. A win for them is a win for us.

As a doctor, if suboptimal care was delivered, ask yourself: Would this have been acceptable for your child, spouse/partner, sibling, parent, friend? A teachable moment.

What can medical students, trainees, or attending surgeons do? When you see a patient or a fellow health care provider being treated unfairly, inform your colleague or a superior—not to accuse but, again, as a teachable moment.

What can *gathered* doctors do? I'm glad to report that during morbidity and mortality conferences, more and more departments of surgery are discussing complicated procedures "objectively," by asking questions such as, "Did bias impact care delivery?" "Did bias impact the outcome?" "Were the social determinants of health addressed for this patient?" These are all learning experiences.

What actions can patients of color take? Historically, they have often felt unseen and unheard; it's time for them to change that. Before your appointment, you might google the condition you think you have (e.g., GERD, gastroesophageal reflux disease), read the suggestions, and write down questions. If the doctor enters the room and never sits down, ask him or her how much time they're allotting you because you have several questions about GERD. If he or she says they have the time, ask them to sit, to lessen your anxiety. You can do this without being confrontational. You're the patient: You deserve to put yourself first. Remember: Without you, the doctor doesn't have a job.

What actions can the family and friends of patients take? The value in accompanying a family member or friend to the doctor cannot be overstated—practically and emotionally. Be that second set of ears and eyes, asking questions, taking notes, vetting the doctor, making sure your loved one is seen and heard. Be a translator, if called upon. When negligence in care occurs, it's important not to be silent.

What action can the hairdresser mentioned in the previous section do to have an impact on her community? Maybe she says to every customer in her chair, "For all my ladies, I'm asking if you've had a recent mammogram/annual checkup." Maybe the hairdresser tells her customers that if they can show that they went to their doctor, their next styling is 20 percent off. She can post flyers about mammography screening. She can supply healthy snacks. She can make her shop a cell phone–free zone, so her clients can unplug and reduce their stress.

What action can the SEPTA bus driver take? Well, they have a daily captive audience of commuters. Perhaps they can procure a small budget to make up signs like the ones at St. Chris to be placed in buses and trains, or signs that ask riders if they're updated on their Covid vaccines, or signs that include facts like, "Black women have a far greater rate of heart disease than other women . . . have you made an appointment to see a cardiologist?"

What action can that single mom take? She needs to take care of herself, so she needs to find local health care providers (or as local as they get) with weekend or nighttime hours—they exist!—so that when she finally gets done at seven o'clock, there's a nearby place to go with appointments until nine. She can schedule a visit even if it's months hence, and let her employer know well in advance.

Action is necessary; so is accountability. We must hold ourselves and each other accountable. I tried to keep my hometown's Department of Public Health accountable to its own mission statement but failed. Rather, I believe they failed. Fortunately, the new health commissioner and I are allies working together for the residents of Philadelphia. If you're not going to live up to your stated purpose, then either change the purpose or get out of the way and let someone else act and lead.

Act in collaboration with those in other industries who share the same mission.

5. SHARE what works and what doesn't.

It's clear that some of the actions we've been taking for years—for decades—are not working. We must stop funding the same organizations, with the same leadership, with the same dead-end ideas resulting in the same lack of measurable improvement, over and over and over, hoping *this time* for different results. A great deal of federal money has gone to state and city health departments, to hospitals and nonprofits and academic institutions, earmarked to help with racial health disparity—and it wasn't spent on that. Or it *was*, yet nothing really changed. Those days need to end. No more money if you can't show measurable improvement.

This progress-free churn will change only if we have elected officials who believe in this vision of health equity. Such change can't be mandated; sure, it can be recommended, but depending on who's in the House and Senate, the possibility of health care–related funding overhaul may end there. That's why so much of the action has to be at the local and state levels. To see impactful government action in our lifetime, we must engage our mayors and governors.

If you're doing something that's having positive impact, please share it with others. So many organizations and groups spend too much time working in silos. Share what you're doing. Share it in peer-reviewed journals and articles. Share it in quarterly meetings. Teach other people what you've done that works. Did your organization with the massive budget operate more effectively once it broke into smaller pieces? At BDCC, I found that it took lots of imagination to succeed on a very limited budget.

Share, because we're dealing with a systemic problem. We want North Philadelphia to improve, and we want the whole city of Philadelphia to improve, but we need all of America to improve.

Find a way to measure your impact. Did things improve because of a reallocation of resources? A new overall strategy? Timing? During the pandemic, timing was a massive problem; had the timing (*urgency*) been different, lives would have been saved, and the virus would not have spread as fast and far. Why did the authorities wait so long to do widespread testing in the highest-positivity zip codes of the city? For any initiative, a key question is: Where do the available resources need to go first to make the greatest impact? Do you ask that each and every time you get money? Does your organization?

I like the old adage, "How do you eat an elephant? One chunk at a time." I mean no disrespect to elephants or to animal lovers. I love animals. As I write this, my dog Carson is curled at my feet. But the point is this: You can't eat an elephant all at once or you'll be eating it forever. When it comes to health care initiatives, we should choose a single, manageably sized chunk of the United States for a test run. Let's apply a limited budget to a limited problem and see what kind of measurable results we get. If we're successful, let's apply the same smart strategies and techniques to other chunks. Sure, there are particulars to every region in the country, but you get the idea. (Many of our concerns for Region 3, the one I oversaw, were the same as those of the other nine, but others—such as maternal mortality and opioid use—were more pressing for us.) If one community-based organization receiving federal funding to address maternal morbidity and mortality and infant mortality is getting exceptional results in St. Louis, say, then let's amplify that model across other cities in other states. If my Center for Health Equity at 2001 W. Lehigh Avenue is getting good results doing things a certain innovative way, then leaders from other cities should come and see who we are and what we're doing and try to emulate that to the extent that they can. I'm convinced that our location—annexed to a church, across the street from a high school, behind public housing, along a bus route, not far from a major academic medical center in the event of escalation of care—is one of the biggest reasons we're thriving. That's a learned lesson that others can take back to their communities.

Gather your data. Do more of what works. Share it with others.

Acknowledge—Believe—Identify—Act—Share

There is no magic pill. Everyone who has suffered from this inequitable system is right to want quicker evidence of markedly improved access, resources, treatment, and especially outcomes. Yet even the best effort will take time to show significant impact.

But we know what's broken so let's go fix it.

Yes, it takes "we," but it also takes "you," the individual. Following a talk I gave on this very subject in the first days of 2023, there was a Q&A session, and a young Black medical student stood at the microphone, wondering what he could do to help.

"You're doing it!" I told him. "Standing there, as a Black man in that white coat, you're doing it! Graduate. Thrive. So that hospitals come to recruit you to their residency. Volunteer. Do not get sucked into the vortex of *You are the face for every little Black boy and Black girl and Latino boy and Latino girl*, which in some ways you *are*, but put the oxygen mask on *you* first. That's what's going to make you a leader. On social media, amplify when you score well on your in-service exam. 'I knocked it out of the park!' That's what you post. 'I matched in my residency!' Post that. 'I did great on my shelf exam!' Post that. Look, I know how much you want to do. But you'll accomplish so much more if you're selfish about the investment in yourself. Put all the energy in you, and do a little bit to helping others. Then, as you build that platform, and you get those degrees behind your name, you'll be able to help so, so much more."

Soon after that talk, I was giving someone else a pep talk: me. I was privileged to oversee a whole region of the country, with a massive budget, yet I felt I could make an even bigger impact if I just focused on my health care center and had the freedom to educate and be a catalyst across the nation. More than anything I wanted to create the best possible situation for the next generation of Philadelphia youth so that they had the best possible outcomes, the best chance at achieving their dreams. My own dream was to build another health center, one focused more squarely on the social determinants of health. I wanted it to include a literacy program and other tutoring. I planned to scour the country for local efforts that had worked well with literacy, on shoestring budgets, and make that a template.

Quietly, I was planning my departure.

27

ENOUGH

On Dr. Martin Luther King Jr. Day of Service, 2023, I attended, with Byron and my sons, an event at Mary McLeod Bethune School, a pre-K–8 school in the Tioga section of Philadelphia. The event was sponsored by TaylorMADE Opportunities and the goal was to find ways to prevent or reduce the rampant violence in neighborhoods like the ones we served during the pandemic, like the one where the school is located, like the one where I grew up. The event also aimed to provide "trauma-informed care" for young kids from these communities. The brave children who volunteered to talk about their experiences were between the ages of ten and seventeen, predominantly Black and predominantly male, though there were girls present as well. All of them had been impacted by the trauma of violence.

Listening to them talk was gut-wrenching. I had to hold back tears. I wasn't the one who had experienced their trauma, so it felt wrong to cry. Who was I to display more grief than these children who had lost their fill-in-the-blank—father, mother, brother, sister, best friend, cousin, uncle, classmate, teammate?

You could hear a pin drop as the kids talked, often in monotones.

One boy spoke of hating Philly and desperately wanting to move out, to do something good in his life, to make a safer place for his mom. Another boy told us that since his stepdad was killed, he had assumed the role of man of the household at the ripe old age of thirteen. Another boy, also thirteen, who had also lost his father to gun violence, said, neither with pride nor shame, that he had joined a particular "group" (the term "gang" is falling out of fashion) because their rival group was the one that killed his dad; this way he could plot and eventually take his revenge.

What a burden for a thirteen-year-old to carry. I sat in the circle of chairs, with my own children, my oldest then fourteen, the twins twelve, so they could listen and understand what twelve and fourteen looks like in a different neighborhood. So they could recognize that they were more similar than they were different. So that they could stay humble and grateful for what they had, and know that they were not "better than." Children have no control over the environments in which they are born. Our home was all of a dozen miles from where these children grew up, but it was another universe.

Most of the young people who spoke wore hand-me-downs of hand-me-downs. Food had been set out—pizza, donuts, juice, mostly carbs and sugar—and for more than a few of the kids it would be their sole meal of the day. The event started at nine o'clock on a Monday morning, a day the schools were closed in honor of Rev. Dr. King's birthday. But these children weren't sleeping in. They were there to be in a "safe space," to have a meal.

Toward the end of the presentation, there was time for closing thoughts from the audience. Community leaders had been invited. There were promises by this leader to mentor that kid, and that leader to mentor this kid; incremental as the effort may have appeared, it made me glad. I'm all for one-on-one. It's an approach that needs to be replicated citywide. Every vulnerable child gets a dedicated adult to help him or her through, whatever it takes.

Afterward, the principal pulled me aside. "We need you to come back," she said. "I know this day turned out to be more about our young boys, but our girls need to see you, too. They never get this close to someone who's achieved what you have."

I probably didn't look like what they imagined a surgeon looks like—not that that was something they ever gave a thought to. I wore my MLK hoodie, black joggers, high-top pink patent leather Jordans. I'd wear that outfit every day if I could. And I thought: *Yeah, I can wear that, and people can have whatever impression they have of me, but I'm board-certified in two surgical specialties, sit on foundation boards, live in a quiet, safe neighborhood with a wide tree-lined street and parks to walk the dog and play in.*

So many people look at these kids and form an instant impression of them, too, certain they're going nowhere, destined for nothing. That they're not worth having hopes and expectations for.

The real problem is that lots of the kids think the same thing. Why wouldn't you, when you've been told it your whole life?

Moments like that are what helped make up my mind. After a year in government, I resigned, in May of 2023. I had learned many valuable lessons there—about health policy, legislation processes, and funding on a federal level. It was a privilege to serve. But I felt I would be more effective in promoting and achieving equity in health care—and I'd be happier, generally—if I were doing it "on the ground and without guard rails." Somewhat confined, I was not maximizing my abilities. In my exit interview, I couldn't help but get in one more plug for the importance of understanding social determinants. "Wealth is linked to homeownership. Homeownership is linked to education. Education is linked to health outcomes, and health outcomes are exacerbated by racial injustice. If we are really talking about achieving health equity, all those things must be addressed, and I could not do all of that within HHS."[1]

Just over a month after my final day there, while walking around my hometown, I found myself, like so many others on the East Coast and in the Midwest, looking up at an eerie, orange sky, a result of the smoke being blown over our part of the country from massive Canadian wildfires. I prayed for all the little children who would have difficulty breathing that day. I knew that misery is not distributed equally. Black children suffer from asthma at a rate more than twice that of white children, so a greater percentage of them will likely suffer when air quality deteriorates. For a long time it was said that one reason for elevated asthma levels in Black children was that their household and community smoked too much. Yet according to the CDC, Black Americans and white Americans smoke at a similar rate; in fact, in eight of the ten years from 2011 to 2020, whites had a higher rate of smoking than Blacks.[2] We must continue to dispel subjective narratives with objective data. The data should drive intervention.

So why do Black kids have more asthma than white kids? Is it yet another unfortunate result of redlining? Of so many highways cutting through Black-dominant cities, toxic waste dumps nearby, poor maintenance of communities where Black Americans lived not by choice but because there was no choice?

A few days later I participated in a learning opportunity for high school girls and women at Dobbins High School, across the street from our health center. The event, titled "Period Poverty," was run by a women's organization and an impressive young high school advocate. Until that day I hadn't encountered the term, but as soon as I heard the advocate describe period poverty—the difficulties and stigma around menstruation but also around being pregnant, valuing your body, sexually transmitted diseases, and intimate partner violence—I realized I had experienced it in my day. It just didn't have a name back then.

Period poverty affects one in four females globally. It's a leading cause of death in young women in the countries where it's most acute. The conversation leaders described how in places like Kenya, Syria, Uganda, Bangladesh, Angola, and others, girls with their periods can't go to school because there are no tampons or maxi pads; they can't return to school until their period stops. I addressed the high school girls in attendance first as a doctor and parent: If they had an issue while in school, I said, then they should go to the teacher or the school nurse, who often has a stash of these items; if that didn't help, then we at the health care center, "literally across the street from you," could supply what they needed.

Then I addressed the girls more intimately, as someone who was once just like them. "I must have been somewhere between sixth and eighth grade, and I didn't always have tampons or pads," I told them. "I recall getting my period in school, and leaking through my clothing, and everyone seeing it, and how embarrassed I felt. I went to the nurse to call my mom, but she couldn't come because she was at work, so she called a family member who happened to be a surgical physician assistant, and she went to the thrift store, bought some clothes, and brought them to school so I could change. I remember how incredibly grateful I felt because just a couple hours before I felt so embarrassed that I wanted to disappear." The memories were flooding back. "Other times at school when I got my period and didn't have pads I would go to the bathroom, take toilet paper or sometimes hard paper towels, which hurt but they were more absorbent, and ball them up and fold them as much as I could and fashion a pad so I wouldn't leak." I told them about the blue jumpsuits we wore back in the day, with elastic around the upper legs in the crotch area, and how I was relieved if I was wearing one of those when I got my period and didn't have pads because the elastic helped keep the paper towels in place better than just a pair of underwear; with the underwear, the paper towels would slide out and I would leak.

As I described the trials of teen Ala to the girls, I started crying. I hadn't thought about any of this since I was their age, going through it. Who knew I and so many girls and young women in the good old U.S. of A. had experienced a version of period poverty? And that so many still were? Tough as it was for me to relive the past, I could see the beautiful faces of the girls in front of me lighting up. My experience—my candor about my experience—resonated with them. In the end, our conversation was about more than period poverty. The teachers, counselors, health care professionals and advocates were all there because of our belief in these girls and young women, in their future, in what they could be.

Yeah, I was once them.

What do you do when you've had a goal your entire life and you reach it? That's where I am now. For as long as I've known what it is to have a dream, mine was to become a doctor. Then the dream became more focused. I wanted to be a surgeon, a pediatric surgeon. It happened.

After twenty-plus years of treating and curing with a scalpel, I find myself on an unexpected path of educating, healing, and advocating. I have come to see that my greatest impact is made not solely with my mind and hands, as a surgeon, but also with my voice and platform. Not long ago I returned to Cincinnati Children's Hospital to give a lecture, and afterward I talked with Dr. Victor Garcia, one of my mentors. He could tell that I was torn about returning to the OR; after all, I had trained for so many years to do just that.

"C. Everett Koop saved way more lives outside of the operating room," he said.

I felt such relief. Dr. Koop had been Dr. Garcia's mentor. Like both of us, Koop was a pediatric surgeon. Then he went on to become the U.S. surgeon general. "So what's next for you, young Jedi?" Dr. Garcia asked me.

I knew I needed to pursue my new course, one that maximized influence on the most lives.

I'm not worried about what's next as long as it's something that beneficially impacts people, particularly children, who have been left behind. That's my greatest passion because I am that child: overlooked but, with proper nurturing, capable of anything. To elevate future greatness in kids when they're young, when they believe they can do anything: It's beautiful. Get them at the right time and they'll grow up believing there's no chance they *won't* achieve what they want.

Maybe I'll go back someday to the operating room. For me, it provides sanctuary, much like a church. It's one of the places where I have found peace.

Whether or not I'm in the OR, there are things about surgery that will never leave me, especially the idea of doing everything you possibly can to succeed. Not accepting "no" for an answer. Being relentless and thorough and unwilling to accept failure.

After each complex operation I performed, my mind was partly, even mostly, back in the OR. I would come home, and even though I was with my loving family, I was silently reviewing every step of the procedure I had just completed. Had all quadrants been inspected? Is his pain controlled? Are her drains putting out? Are they secure? Did I miss anything? Did I do everything I could? Even when I finally lay my head on the pillow—maybe especially then—I was still thinking about it.

What new, creative, effective ways can we address entrenched inequity and ensure that this time—*this time*—we finally get it right? For me, each night I put my head on my pillow, I'll be wondering:

Was there anything I missed? Did we do everything we could? God willing, is it enough?

Acknowledgments

This is all surreal. Like so many of you, my life turned upside down during Covid. I did not anticipate that by helping my fellow citizens my life would evolve into following a totally different path.

My life has been spared more than once, and I am grateful to God. I continue to walk by faith and not by sight as He orders my steps.

To my husband, Byron, thank you for being right by my side with your honest critique, saying things I need to hear, not always what I want to hear.

To my children, Ellison, Robeson, and Langston, you are all unique. My love for you is infinite and I can't wait to see what you do next. Please know that if your mind can conceive it, you can achieve it. Continue to compete with yourself, setting and raising your own bar.

To my parents, I appreciate you. I am grateful to you. Mom: You sacrificed your childhood for us. I know you did the best you could with what you had. You deserve to live your best life right now. Dad: Living for years with incurable cancer takes courage. Continue to look for light even on dark days. You have my love and everything you need to be comfortable.

To my brother, Kamau, my Day One, this life is not a dress rehearsal. Live every day on purpose, without regret.

To my grandmother, the original Dr. Stanford, thank you for what you are to our family and what you have been to the city of Philadelphia.

To Maya, Myles, and Byron Jr., continue to thrive. It's wonderful to have a front row seat to your life as a bonus mom.

To Mama Drayton, your prayers avail much. Thank you.

To my extended family and friends, thanks for continuing to pick up the phone when I call. You know my door is always open to you.

To all my Sorors of Alpha Kappa Alpha Sorority, Incorporated, we continue to be in Service to All Mankind.

To the Senegalese women at Amy's Hair Braiding on Ogontz Avenue, thank you for keeping my hair on point! I valued those hours. It was protected time.

To all my teachers and mentors, thank you for investing in me.

To the amazing team of volunteers, administrative staff, doctors, nurses, and clinical folks of the Black Doctors Consortium, you see what we did? Never underestimate the power of one, or how strong the collective can be.

To all the churches, and especially my home church of Salem Baptist Church of Abington, that opened their sanctuaries and parking lots to us, fed us, and prayed for us, thank you.

To Andrew Postman, thank you for your attention to detail with my book, your skillful way with words, and most important, your patience with needed pauses and tears as we got through the tough parts.

To Jennifer Weis, thank you for getting a first-time author a book deal. To LaSharah Bunting, thanks for seeing the potential. To Ian Straus and all the folks at Simon & Schuster, thank you for your help in so many ways.

Life is about experiences. The older you get, the fewer new ones you get to have. This has been a ride!

Notes

Chapter 1: Prep

1. "Flint Official Resigns After Using Racial Slur to Talk About Water Crisis," *Time*, June 5, 2017. https://time.com/4806646/flint-michigan-water-crisis-racial-slur/.
2. "Life Expectancy in the United States," Www.everycrsreport.com, n.d. https://www.everycrsreport.com/reports/RL32792.html#_Toc194633794.
3. "What Is Driving Widening Racial Disparities in Life Expectancy?," KFF, May 23, 2023. https://www.kff.org/racial-equity-and-health-policy/issue-brief/what-is-driving-widening-racial-disparities-in-life-expectancy/.
4. "Study: Black Kids More Likely to Die After Surgery than White Kids," STAT, July 20, 2020. https://www.statnews.com/2020/07/20/healthy-black-children-more-likely-die-surgery/.
5. "Positive Tests Higher in Poorer Neighborhoods Despite Six Times More Testing in Higher-Income Neighborhoods, Researcher Says," Drexel University Dornsife School of Public Health, April 7, 2020. https://drexel.edu/dornsife/news/in-the-media/2020/April/postive-tests-higher-in-poorer-areas/.
6. "Only 5.7% of US Doctors Are Black, and Experts Warn the Shortage Harms Public Health—National Medical Association," Www.nmanet.org., n.d. https://www.nmanet.org/news/632592/Only-5.7-of-US-doctors-are-Black-and-experts-warn-the-shortage-harms-public-health.htm.
7. Simar Singh Bajaj, Lucy Tu, and Fatima Cody Stanford, "Superhuman, but Never Enough: Black Women in Medicine," *The Lancet* 398 (10309) (2021): 1398–99. https://doi.org/10.1016/s0140-6736(21)02217-0.
8. "New International Study: U.S. Health System Ranks Last Among 11 Countries; Many Americans Struggle to Afford Care as Income Inequality Widens," www.commonwealthfund.org, August 4, 2021. https://commonwealthfund

.org/press-release/2021/new-international-study-us-health-system-ranks-last
-among-11-countries-many.s

Chapter 4: College and Cadavers

1. Valerie Strauss, "Perspective: What You Need to Know About Standardized Testing," *Washington Post*, February 1, 2021. https://www.washingtonpost.com/education/2021/02/01/need-to-know-about-standardized-testing/.

Chapter 5: The Source of Our Own River

1. "Unequal Treatment: What Health Care System Administrators Need to Know About Racial and Ethnic Disparities in Healthcare," Institute of Medicine, March 2022. https://nap.nationalacademies.org/resource/10260/disparities_admin.pdf.
2. "Black Men Make Up Less than 3% of Physicians. That Requires Immediate Action, Say Leaders in Academic Medicine," AAMC, n.d., accessed November 3, 2023. https://www.aamc.org/news/black-men-make-less-3-physicians-requires-immediate-action-say-leaders-academic-medicine.
3. Usha Lee McFarling, "In Counties with More Black Doctors, Black People Live Longer, 'Astonishing' Study Finds," STAT, April 14, 2023. https://www.statnews.com/2023/04/14/black-doctors-primary-care-life-expectancy-mortality/.

Chapter 10: Levels of Care

1. Claire Miller, Sarah Kliff, and Larry Buchanan, "Childbirth Is Deadlier for Black Families Even When They're Rich, Expansive Study Finds," *New York Times*, "The Upshot," February 12, 2023.https://www.nytimes.com/interactive/2023/02/12/upshot/child-maternal-mortality-rich-poor.html.

Chapter 11: Outcomes I Didn't Count On

1. "Race Is a Risk Factor for Postoperative Death in Apparently Healthy Children in United States," www.nationwidechildrens.org, n.d. https://www.nationwidechildrens.org/newsroom/news-releases/2020/07/race-is-risk-factor-for-postoperative-death-study.

Chapter 14: Invisible Men and Women

1. Yance Ford, *The Color of Care*, Harpo Productions, 2022.

Chapter 15: Black Doctors

1. "U.S. Poverty Rate: Top 25 Most Populated Cities 2019," Statista, September 2020. https://www.statista.com/statistics/205637/percentage-of-poor-people-in-the-top-20-most-populated-cities-in-the-us/.
2. "COVID-19 More Prevalent, Deadlier in U.S. Counties with Higher Black

Populations," Www.commonwealthfund.org, n.d. https://www.common
wealthfund.org/blog/2020/covid-19-more-prevalent-deadlier-us-counties
-higher-black-populations.

3. Marcela Isaza, "Sean Penn Wants to 'Save Lives' with Free Drive-thru Coronavirus Testing in California," *USA Today*, accessed November 3, 2023. https://
www.usatoday.com/story/entertainment/celebrities/2020/04/10/sean-penn
-wants-save-lives-free-coronavirus-testing-california/5135081002/.

4. "Unequal Treatment: What Healthcare Providers Need to Know About Racial
and Ethnic Disparities in Health Care," 2002. https://nap.nationalacademies
.org/resource/10260/disparities_providers.pdf.

5. Usha Lee McFarling, "In Counties with More Black Doctors, Black People
Live Longer, 'Astonishing' Study Finds," STAT, April 14, 2023. https://www
.statnews.com/2023/04/14/black-doctors-primary-care-life-expectancy-mor
tality/.

Chapter 17: Where's the Money?

1. Sean Collins Walsh, *Inquirer*, "Council Implores Kenney Administration to
Support Black Doctors COVID-19 Consortium," https://www.inquirer.com.
May 27, 2020. https://www.inquirer.com/news/funding-black-doctors-covid
-19-consortium-mayor-jim-kenney-cherelle-parker-20200527.html.

2. Ibid.

3. Ibid.

4. Ed Pilkington, "Black Americans Dying of Covid-19 at Three Times the Rate
of White People," *The Guardian*, "World News," May 20, 2020. https://www
.theguardian.com/world/2020/may/20/black-americans-death-rate-covid
-19-coronavirus.

Chapter 18: Moving the Needle

1. "Covid Death Rate Among Black Children Nearly Three Times Higher than
White Kids," Bloomberg.com, March 14, 2023. https://www.bloomberg.com
/news/articles/2023-03-14/covid-killed-black-children-three-times-more
-often-than-white-children#xj4y7vzkg.

Chapter 19: False Narrative, Real Scam

1. Shao Lin et al., "COVID-19 Symptoms and Deaths Among Healthcare Workers, United States," *Emerging Infectious Diseases Journal*, CDC 28, no. 4 (August
2022), wwwnc.cdc.gov. https://doi.org/10.3201/eid2808.212200.

2. Juliana Feliciano Reyes, Ellie Silverman, Ellie Rushing, and Oona Goodin-
Smith, *Inquirer*, "The City Trusted a Group of College Kids . . ." https://www
.inquirer.com/health/coronavirus/philly-fighting-covid-vaccine-fighting-an
drei-doroshin-20210131.html.

3. Max Marin, "Philly Vaccine Map: Richer Neighborhoods Are Getting

More Doses," Billy Penn at WHYY, March 11, 2021. https://billypenn
.com/2021/03/11/philadelphia-vaccine-map-zip-distribution-racial-inequity
-neighborhoods/.

4. "Philly's Vaccine Supply Flowing to Some Suburbs 4 Times Faster than City
Neighborhoods," WHYY, n.d., accessed November 3, 2023. https://whyy.org
/articles/phillys-vaccine-supply-flowing-to-some-wealthy-suburbs-4-times
-faster-than-many-city-neighborhoods/.

5. Marin, "Philly Vaccine Map: Richer Neighborhoods Are Getting More Doses."

Chapter 21: Our Own

1. Melissa Romero, "What's the Life Expectancy of Your Zip Code?," *Curbed
Philly*, April 7, 2016. https://philly.curbed.com/2016/4/7/11380408/life-ex
pectancy-in-philly-neighborhoods.

2. Christopher J. Peterson, Benjamin Lee, and Kenneth Nugent, "Covid-19 Vaccination Hesitancy Among Healthcare Workers—A Review." https://www
.mdpi.com/2076-393X/10/6/948; Judith Green-McKenzie, Frances S. Shofer,
Florence Momplaisir, et al., "Factors Associated with Covid-19 Vaccine Re-
ceipt by Health Care Personnel at a Major Academic Hospital During the
First Months of Vaccine Availability." https://jamanetwork.com/journals/jama
networkopen/fullarticle/2786699.

Chapter 23: The Kids

1. Bhavini Patel Murthy, "COVID-19 Vaccination Coverage Among Ado-
lescents Aged 12–17 Years—United States, December 14, 2020–July 31,
2021," MMWR, Morbidity and Mortality Weekly Report 70. https://doi
.org/10.15585/mmwr.mm7035e1.

Chapter 24: Owning It

1. "Cardiac Arrest Deaths Are Rising—Especially Among Younger Black Adults,"
n.d. Www.heart.org. https://www.heart.org/en/news/2020/11/10/cardiac-ar
rest-deaths-are-rising-especially-among-younger-black-adults.

2. Ibid.

Chapter 25: The Social Determinants of Health

1. "Pennsylvania's School Funding System Is Unconstitutional, Judge Says,"
WHYY, n.d. https://whyy.org/articles/pennsylvania-school-funding-lawsuit
-judge-rules-unconstitutional/.

2. Emma Garcia, "Schools Are Still Segregated, and Black Children Are Paying a
Price," Economic Policy Institute, February 12, 2020. https://www.epi.org/pub
lication/schools-are-still-segregated-and-black-children-are-paying-a-price/.

3. National Center for Education Statistics, "COE—College Enrollment Rates,"

Nces.ed.gov, May 2022. https://nces.ed.gov/programs/coe/indicator/cpb/col lege-enrollment-rate.

4. Melanie Hanson, "College Enrollment Statistics [2020]: Total + by Demographic," Education Data Initiative, July 26, 2022. https://educationdata.org /college-enrollment-statistics.

5. Sara Weissman, "Black Enrollment Declines, Gaps Increase," Inside Higher Ed., n.d., accessed November 3, 2023. https://insidehighered.com /news/2022/09/21/black-community-college-students-face-stark-disparities.

6. "Why Is Black Male Enrollment in Decline? | BestColleges," www.bestcol leges.com, n.d., accessed November 3, 2023. https://bestcolleges.com/blog /black-male-enrollment/.

7. Emily Peterson, "Racial Inequality in Public School Discipline for Black Students in the United States," Ballard Brief, 2021. https://ballardbrief.byu.edu /issue-briefs/racial-inequality-in-public-school-discipline-for-black-students -in-the-united-states.

8. "The Failure Cycle Causing a Shortage of Black Male Teachers," *PBS News-Hour*, January 6, 2017. https://pbs.org/newshour/show/failure-cycle-causing -shortage-black-male-teachers.

9. Editor, "The Black Percentage of School Principals Has Declined in Recent Years," *The Journal of Blacks in Higher Education*, January 9, 2023. https://www .jbhe.com/2023/01/the-black-percentage-of-school-principals-has-declined -in-recent-years/.

10. "Unequal Treatment: What Health Care System Administrators Need to Know About Racial and Ethnic Disparities in Healthcare," Institute of Medicine, March 2022. https://nap.nationalacademies.org/resource/10260/dispari ties_admin.pdf.

11. "Gaslighting of Black Medical Trainees Makes Residency Something to 'Survive,'" STAT, March 10, 2022. https://www.statnews.com/2022/03/10/gas lighting-black-medical-trainees-residency/.

12. Mytien Nguyen et al., "Association of Sociodemographic Characteristics with US Medical Student Attrition," *JAMA Internal Medicine*, July. https://doi .org/10.1001/jamainternmed.2022.2194.

Chapter 26: We Know What's Broken. Now Let's Fix It.

1. Latoya Hill, Nambi Ndugga, and Samantha Artiga. "Key Data on Health and Health Care by Race and Ethnicity," KFF, March 15, 2023. https://kff.org /racial-equity-and-health-policy/report/key-data-on-health-and-health-care -by-race-and-ethnicity/.

2. Ibid.

3. Ibid.

4. Risa Lavizzo-Mourey and David Williams, "Being Black Is Bad for Your

Health," *U.S. News & World Report*, 2016. https://www.usnews.com/opinion/blogs/policy-dose/articles/2016-04-14/theres-a-huge-health-equity-gap-between-whites-and-minorities.

5. Carolyn B. Swope, Diana Hernández, and Lara J. Cushing, "The Relationship of Historical Redlining with Present-Day Neighborhood Environmental and Health Outcomes: A Scoping Review and Conceptual Model," *Journal of Urban Health* 99, no. 6 (2022). https://doi.org/10.1007/s11524-022-00665-z.

6. Nambi Ndugga and Samantha Artiga, "Disparities in Health and Health Care: 5 Key Questions and Answers," KFF, April 21, 2023. https://kff.org/racial-equity-and-health-policy/issue-brief/disparities-in-health-and-health-care-5-key-question-and-answers/.

7. Ibid.

Chapter 27: Enough

1. Aubrey Whelan, "Ala Stanford Steps Down from a Federal Health Position to Focus Efforts in Philadelphia," https://www.inquirer.com, May 9, 2023. https://inquirer.com/health/ala-stanford-stepping-down-health-and-human-services-health-equity-philadelphia-20230509.html.

2. René A. Arrazola, "US Cigarette Smoking Disparities by Race and Ethnicity—Keep Going and Going!," *Preventing Chronic Disease* 20, 2023. https://doi.org/10.5888/pcd20.220375.

About the Author

DR. ALA STANFORD is founder of the Black Doctors Consortium, a national leader in health equity, a health care policy advisor, and former regional director of the U.S. Department of Health and Human Services of the mid-Atlantic region appointed by President Biden. In May 2024 she was appointed Professor of Practice in Biology at the University of Pennsylvania with two additional appointments in the Perelman School of Medicine and Annenberg School for Communication. A practicing physician for more than twenty years and founder of R.E.A.L. Concierge Medicine, Dr. Stanford is board-certified by the American Board of Surgery in both pediatric and adult general surgery, and she serves as a medical and health correspondent for national media outlets. Dr. Stanford gained international recognition during the Covid-19 pandemic for using the infrastructure of her pediatric surgery practice to create a grassroots organization focused on education, testing, contact tracing, and vaccination in communities lacking access to care and resources. She and her team provided direct care for hundreds of thousands as well as for countless others nationwide through her organization's messaging. She subsequently opened a multidisciplinary ambulatory care center bearing her name in a neighborhood in Philadelphia with one of the lowest life expectancies in the city.

Dr. Stanford has received many awards and honors, including being named a Top 10 CNN Hero, one of *Fortune* magazine's "World's 50 Greatest Leaders," and one of *Forbes's* Most Influential Women. She has also received the American College of Surgeons 2023 Domestic Surgical Volunteerism Award and the George H. W. Bush Points of Light Award. She was selected for the 2024 Distinguished Alumni from The Pennsylvania State University, and the City of Philadelphia commissioned a street in her name. She lives in the suburbs of Philadelphia with her husband and children.